Operative Dentistry in the Phantom Lab

Dr. Fahad Alqahtani

ISBN
978-1-5437-4910-6 (hc)
978-1-5437-4816-1 (sc)
978-1-5437-4817-8 (e)

Library of Congress Control Number: 2018959943

Print information available on the last page.

To order additional copies of this book, contact
Toll Free 800 101 2657 (Singapore)
Toll Free 1 800 81 7340 (Malaysia)
www.partridgepublishing.com/singapore
orders.singapore@partridgepublishing.com

03/16/2019

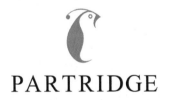

PARTRIDGE

CONTENTS

INTRODUCTION

It is important for dental students to practice treatments on phantom lab heads and ivory teeth before practicing in a real patient's mouth, but most students find it difficult to correlate between a real patient and the tasks performed on ivory teeth.

Dental simulators provide simulated treatments in various training areas, such as restorative dentistry and prosthetics.

Simulating units are not available in all dental colleges all around the world because of the high expense.

This book will help to simulate the operative dental cases for dental students and their supervisors in the phantom lab.

The book is a reference for operative dentistry in the phantom lab; it includes more than eight hundred high-resolution images, illustrations, and tables. Students in preclinical phantom lab sessions will get used to the tools and instruments used in operative dentistry.

The common terms used in operative dentistry are explained with clear and simple images and illustrations. Simulating systems for caries lesions are shown in the phantom lab and their corresponding restorative treatments. Radiographic images and clinical photos are included in the book to help students make the correct caries lesions diagnosis.

Exposing students to real radiographic and clinical images in the phantom lab makes them familiar and ready to treat the real patient in the clinical sessions.

The book describes easy techniques, such as practical step-by-step rubber dam techniques as well as matrix band, retainer application, and teeth preparation and their corresponding restorations with amalgam or composite restoration.

The book saves time and money reduces the effort for dental institutes and faculty members. It also offers new and practical way for the phantom lab assessment exams.

ACKNOWLEDGEMENTS

In the name of God, the Most Gracious, the Most Merciful.

Great thanks to our great creator, our Almighty God, Allah, the author of knowledge and wisdom, who made this book possible.

I would like to express gratitude and sincere appreciation to various people who contribute to the beginning of the book idea and to its completion.

To all the staff of Moustashark Advanced Dental Centre in Riyadh City, who provided the book with valuable photograph images.

To Mr. Khalid Saad, CEO of the center, Ms. Maris Estella Capoy, Ms. Edelyn Tolentino, Ms. Ruby Mei Pisan, and most especially to Ms. Charisse Dimple Dumdumaya, the centre's head nurse, for their great effort and valued participation.

Special thanks to my best adviser and friend, Mr. Mohammed Alqahtani.

Sincere gratitude to Mr. Oqba Alkhuzam, my book designer and editor. Thank you for making the book stunning in order to capture the attention of readers.

Great thanks to my collages in Riyadh Dental College.

To Professor Abdullah Alshamari, the dean of the college, for his full support at the beginning of this journey, which started 2007.

To Dr. Basil Yousef Alamasi, my colleague in the phantom lab sessions, for his support and great participation.

Finally, great thanks to my family: my parents, my wife, and my daughters and sons, who always pray for my success and my inspiration and give me full support and constant love.

1

NUMBERING SYSTEM

Universal System

Primary Teeth														
Upper Right								Upper Left						
			A	B	C	D	E	F	G	H	I	J		
			T	S	R	Q	P	O	N	M	L	K		
Lower Right								Lower Left						

Permanent Teeth															
Upper Right								Upper Left							
1	2	3	4	5	6	7	8	9	10	11	12	13	14	15	16
32	31	30	29	28	27	26	25	24	23	22	21	20	19	18	17
Lower Right								Lower Left							

Universal System

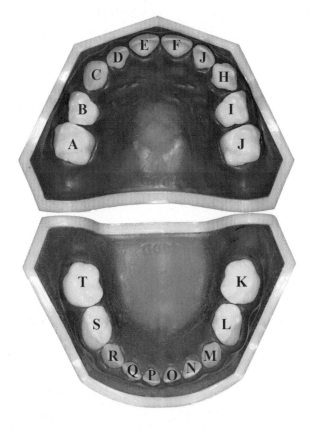
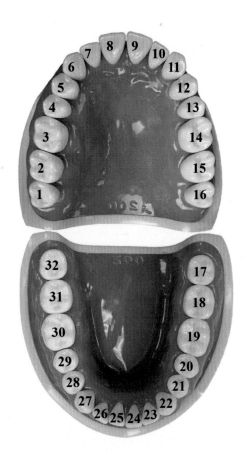

FDI Numbering System

Primary Teeth													
Upper Right							Upper Left						
			55	54	53	52	51	61	62	63	64	65	
			85	84	83	82	81	71	72	73	74	75	
Lower Right							Lower Left						

Permanent teeth															
Upper Right								Upper Left							
18	17	16	15	14	13	12	11	21	22	23	24	25	26	27	28
48	47	46	45	44	43	42	41	31	32	33	34	35	36	37	38
Lower Right								Lower Left							

FDI Numbering System

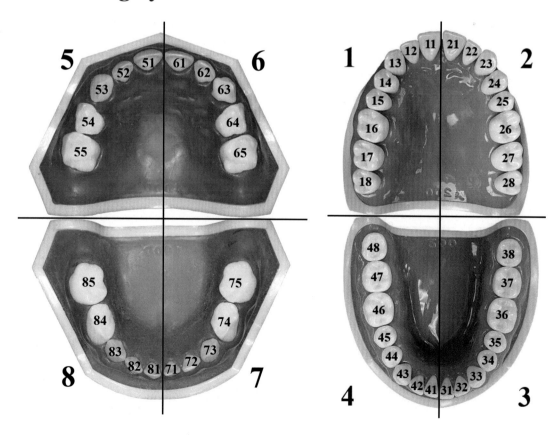

Palmer Numbering System

This system consists of a symbol (⌐ ⌐ ⌐ ⌐) indicating the quadrants in the mouth.

And the numbers and letters indicate the tooth in the quadrant for both primary and permanent teeth.

Primary Teeth													
Upper Right							**Upper Left**						
			e⌋	d⌋	c⌋	b⌋	a⌋	⌊a	⌊b	⌊c	⌊d	⌊e	
			e⌉	d⌉	c⌉	b⌉	a⌉	⌈a	⌈b	⌈c	⌈d	⌈e	
Lower Right							**Lower Left**						

Permanent teeth															
Upper Right								**Upper Left**							
8⌋	7⌋	6⌋	5⌋	4⌋	3⌋	2⌋	1⌋	⌊1	⌊2	⌊3	⌊4	⌊5	⌊6	⌊7	⌊8
8⌉	7⌉	6⌉	5⌉	4⌉	3⌉	2⌉	1⌉	⌈1	⌈2	⌈3	⌈4	⌈5	⌈6	⌈7	⌈8
Lower Right								**Lower Left**							

Palmer Numbering System

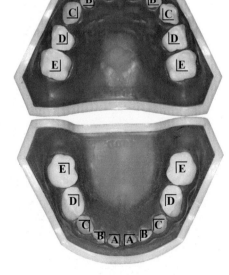
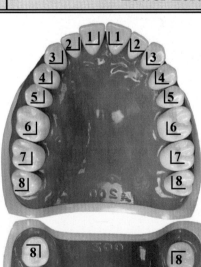
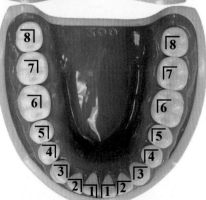

REFERENCES

1. Blinkhorn, A., Choi, C., Paget, H. (1998), "An investigation into the use of the FDI tooth notation system by dental schools in the UK". *Eur J Dent Educ.* 2 (1): 39–41.
2. Harris, Edward F. (2005), "Tooth-Coding Systems in the Clinical Dental Setting." *Dental Anthropology* 18 (2): 44.
3. Havale, R., Sheetal, B. S., Patil, R., Hemant Kumar, R., Anegundi, R. T., Inushekar, K. R. (2015), "Dental notation for primary teeth: A review and suggestion of a novel system." *European Journal of Paediatric Dentistry.* 16 (2): 163–166.
4. Huszár, G. (1989), "The role of the life and works of Adolf Zsigmondy and Ottó Zsigmondy in the history of dentistry." *Fogorv Sz.* 82 (12): 357–63.
5. ISO-3950. "Dentistry: Designation system for teeth and areas of the oral cavity," 4th edition, Document Center Inc., March 15, 2016.
6. Ferguson, J. W. (2005), "The Palmer notation system and its use with personal computer applications." *British Dental Journal,* 198 (9): 551–3.
7. Ross, Michael H., Pawlina, Wojciech (2016), *Histology: A Text and Atlas: With Correlated Cell and Molecular Biology,* Seventh Edition. Wolters Kluwer Health.
8. "Tooth Numbering Systems." Oral Health Topics A–Z. American Dental Association. Archived from the original on November 2, 2006. Retrieved May 26, 2014 (www.archive.org link).

2

DENTAL HANDPIECES AND ROTARY INSTRUMENTS

Dental Handpieces

This instrument holds various disks, cups, or burs, in order to prepare, cut, finish, contour, clean, or polish the tooth or restoration surface.

Handpieces may be powered by electric motor or air turbines and are characterised as high-speed or low-speed, depending on their rotational speed, measured in revolutions per minute (RPMs). This is the frequency of rotation of the handpiece, specifically the number of rotations around a fixed axis in one minute.

Types of Dental Handpieces

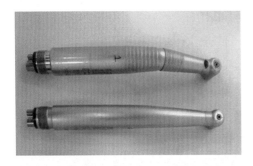

High-Speed Handpiece

Used when planning to cut or remove hard tissue (e.g., tooth structure or restorations or any other dental treatments), designed to permit rotational speeds up to 400,000 RPM. Must be run with water to cool the tooth during preparation to prevent pulpal damage.

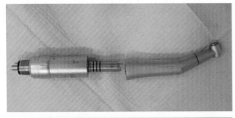

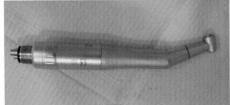

Low-Speed Handpiece

An electric or air-powered handpiece that operates at more than 100,000 RPM.

Used in dental treatments that need less power and speed, such as teeth prophylaxis removal of deep carries and polishing restorations and tooth surfaces.

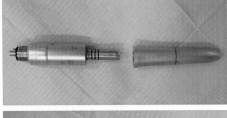

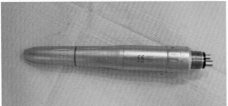

Straight Handpiece

This tool can run up to 40,000 RPM and is used in dental surgery procedures or can be used extra-orally at chairside or in the laboratory for prosthetic appliances and denture adjustment.

Rotary Instruments

These instrument enable dental health professionals to remove, contour, reduce, or shape the tooth structure or dental materials during various dental procedures.

There are two types of rotary dental instruments: burs and finishing and polishing instruments

1. Burs

Dental burs are used in conjunction with the dentist's handpiece for cutting hard tooth or bone tissues or hard restorative materials. There are a huge range of burs made of tungsten carbide or diamond grit, with different shapes and sizes to suit different situations and procedures.

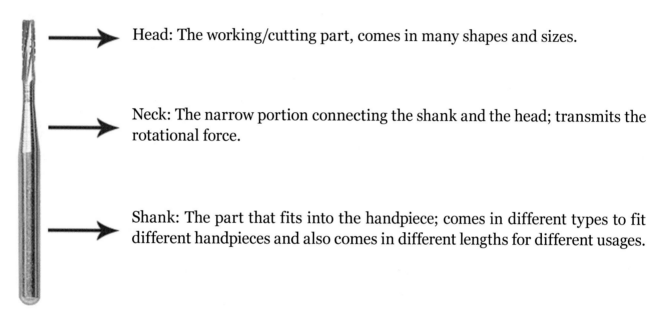

Head: The working/cutting part, comes in many shapes and sizes.

Neck: The narrow portion connecting the shank and the head; transmits the rotational force.

Shank: The part that fits into the handpiece; comes in different types to fit different handpieces and also comes in different lengths for different usages.

Shank Types

Latch-Type Shank (RA)

Fits in low-speed handpieces and contra angles. Latch-type shanks are often available with the same shapes and head design as friction-grip shanks.

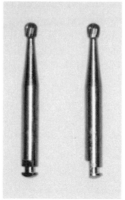
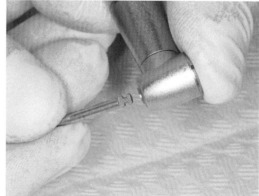

Friction-Grip Shank (FG)

Friction grips are used in conjunction with carbide and diamond head burs. Friction grips are used with high-speed handpieces.

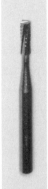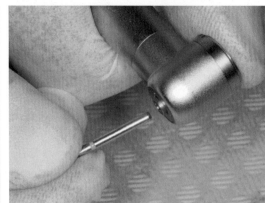

Long Straight Shank (HP)

Long straight shanks are used on slow-speed handpieces, most commonly used for diamond cutting discs. Long straight shanks are also used in surgery procedures and burs.

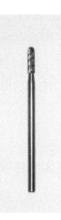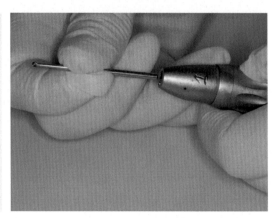

Head Design of Bur

Bladed bur: To cut meta-based restorations or sectioning cast metal copings or crowns.

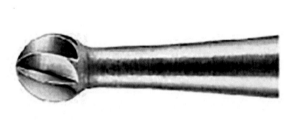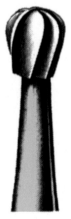

Manufacturing Materials

- steel
- tungsten carbide

Blade Numbers of the Bur

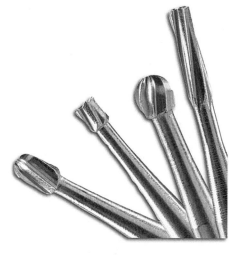 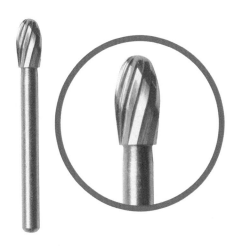

Cutting and preparation are
done using 6–8 blades.

Finishing and polishing is better
using 12, 24, and 30 blades.

Head Shapes of Bur

Round Burs

These are used for caries excavation and cavity preparation. Smaller sizes are often used for single surface cavities; medium sizes are often used for interproximal cavities in anterior teeth.

US No.	1/4	1/2	1	2	3	4	5	6	8
Diameter (mm)	0.5	0.70	0.80	1.00	1.20	1.40	1.50	1.80	2.30

Flat Taper Fissure Bur

These are used for producing a preparation with tapered, divergent walls and a flat floor. Also used for inlay/onlay preparation and to section teeth and cut bone.

US No.	169	170	171
Diameter (mm)	0.90	1.00	1.20

Straight Fissure Burs

These are used for producing preparations with straight parallel sides and flat floors, gaining access to carious dentin, establishing preparation form, and creating retentive locks.

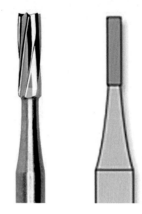

US No.	56	57	58
Diameter (mm)	0.90	1.00	1.20

Inverted Cone Burs

These are used for producing undercuts in cavity preparations; slightly rounded edges on the blade corners reduce chipping for a smoother cut. Ideal for amalgam removal; may also be used for flattening pulpal and gingival walls.

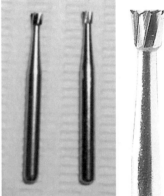

US No.	33.5	34	35	36	37	38	39	41
Diameter(mm)	0.50	0.70	0.80	1.00	1.20	1.40	1.60	1.80

Pear-Shaped Burs

These are used for contouring the occlusal anatomy, preparing cavities, and removing amalgam. Produces an undercut preparation with round internal line angles.

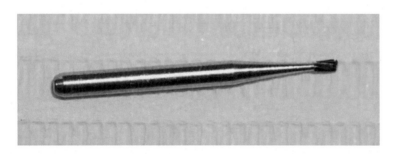

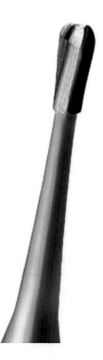

US No.	329	330	331	332
Diameter (mm)	0.60	0.80	1.00	1.20

Abrasive Bur

Diamond nonbladed burs used to shave and cut or prepare the tooth surface or restoration.

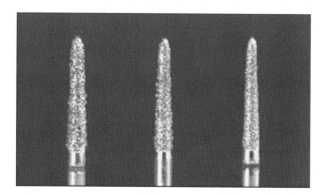

2. Finishing and Polishing Instruments

These are generally used in a low-speed handpiece to finish, polish, or reshape dental material or tooth surfaces to improve their aesthetic quality. These include discs, strips, cups, points, and mounted and unmounted stones. There are three main materials that these instruments are made of: aluminum oxide, silicon carbide, and diamond grit.

Types of Finishing and Polishing Instruments

Diamonds: Finishing diamonds are used to contour, adjust, and smooth composites or porcelain.

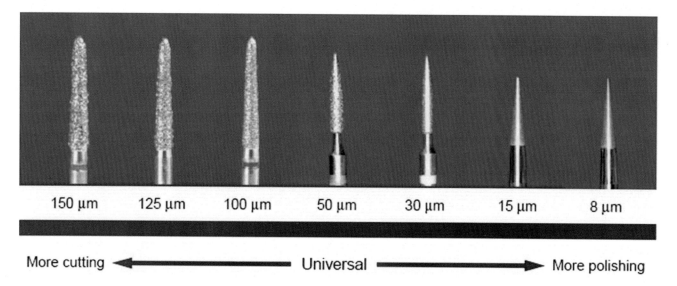

Colour	Grit
Yellow	Ultra-Fine
Red	Fine
Blue	Regular/Medium
Green	Coarse
Black	Super Coarse

Carbide Burs

The most commonly used burs range from 8 to 30 fluted blades

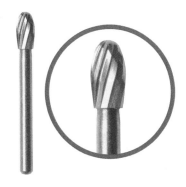

Stones

are used for contouring and finishing restorations, and where maximum abrasion is needed, such as adjusting the occlusion. They do not leave a glossy finish, and it is difficult to achieve refined tooth anatomy.

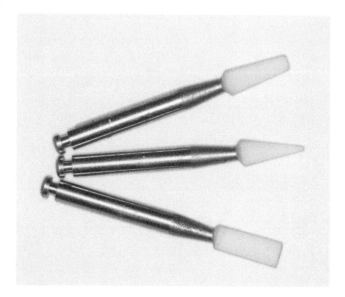

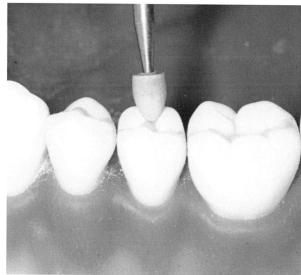

Discs

Finishing and polishing discs are used for gross reduction, contouring, finishing, and polishing restorations. Discs have the reputation of providing the highest polish. Most are coated with an aluminium oxide abrasive. They are used in a sequence of grits, starting with a coarser grit disc and finishing with a superfine grit.

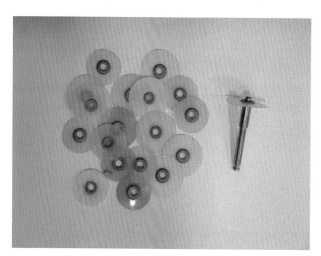

Rubber Wheels, Cups, and Points

Rubber polishing instruments are used to smooth and polish restorative materials.

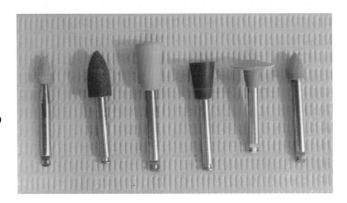

Strips

Mylar Finishing and Polishing Strips

These tools finish and polish the interproximal area of the restorations or tooth structure. The abrasive strips are made of flexible polyester and firmly coated with aluminium oxide particles. They are available in different widths, and they are colour-coded for grit sizes.

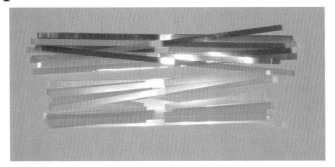

Diamond Finishing and Polishing Strips

These tools are for interproximal finishing and polishing of all materials. Strips allow easy access and precise manual enamel reduction, resulting in a smooth, natural finish. They are made of stainless steel to resist breaking and stretching. Perforated strips are also available and they are colour coded for grit selection. Available in double- or single-sided for more finishing control.

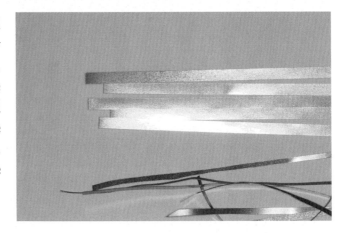

REFERENCES

1. Robinson, Debbie S., Bird, Doni L. (2017), *Modern Dental Assisting* 11th edition, Elsevier.
2. Heymann, Harald O., Swift, Edward J., and Ritter, Andre V. (2013), *Sturdevant's Art & Science of Operative Dentistry,* 6th edition, Elsevier.
3. Boyd, Linda Bartolomucci, (2017), *Dental Instruments: A Pocket Guide*, 6th Edition, Elsevier.
4. Gladwinand, M., and Bagby, M. (2018), *Clinical Aspects of Dental Materials: Theory, Practice, and Cases* 5th edition, Wolters Kluwer.
5. Garg, Nisha, Garg, Amit (2013), *Textbook of Operative Dentistry*, 2nd edition, Jaypee Brothers Medical Publishers.
6. Hilton, Thomas J., Ferracane, Jack L., Broome, James C. (2013), *Summitt's Fundamentals of Operative Dentistry: A Contemporary Approach*, 4th edition, Quintessence Publishing Co.
7. http://www.johnsonpromident.com

3

HAND INSTRUMENTS IN OPERATIVE DENTISTRY

Instruments that are used manually, without a power
source, can be categorised into three groups:

1. Examination instruments
2. Cutting instruments
3. Noncutting instruments

All hand instruments share the same parts: working end, shank, and handle.

Hand Instrument Parts

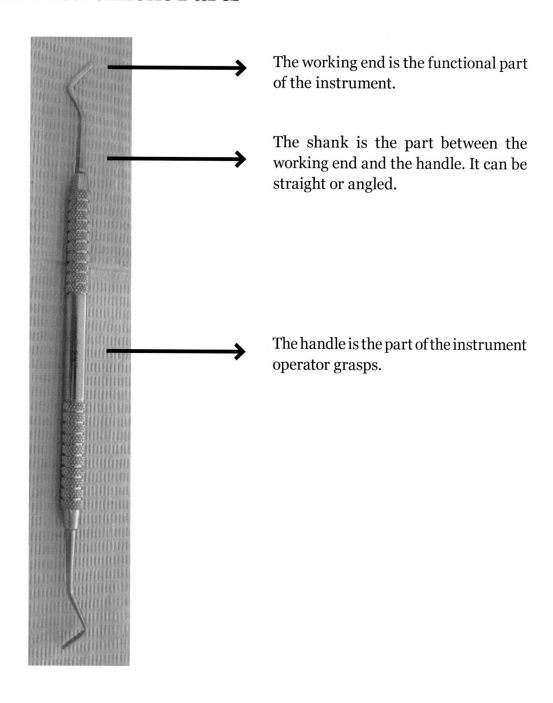

The working end is the functional part of the instrument.

The shank is the part between the working end and the handle. It can be straight or angled.

The handle is the part of the instrument operator grasps.

The working end
can be pointed

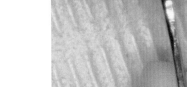

a sharp end to explore
and examine

a blade

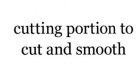

cutting portion to
cut and smooth

or a nib working end

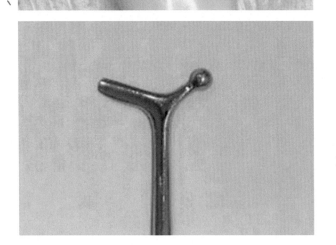

blunt, serrated, or
smooth for packing
or smoothening the
restorative materials.

1. Examination Instruments

Diagnostic Instruments

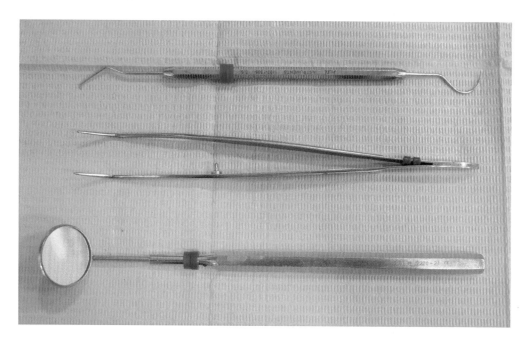

Mouth Mirror

- provides indirect vision
- reflects light for extra illumination
- for retraction and protection of oral tissues

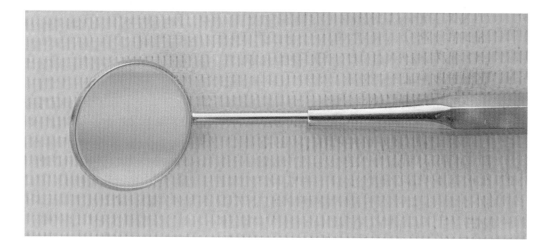

Explorer

- examination of the tooth structure for any defects or areas of decay
- examination of restorations to check for faulty margins or fractures
- removal of excess materials (e.g., cements, liners, and bases)

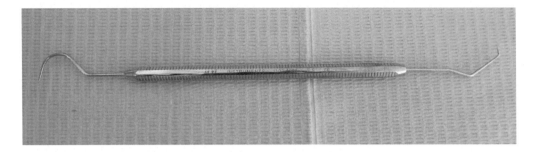

Periodontal Probe

The tip is calibrated in millimetres to measure the depth of periodontal pockets.

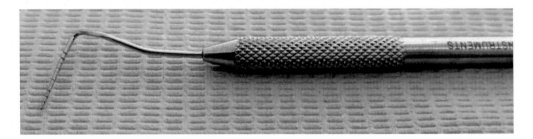

Cotton Pliers (Tweezers)

Used for placing small objects in the mouth and retrieving small objects from the mouth or to pass cotton or other material to the dentist.

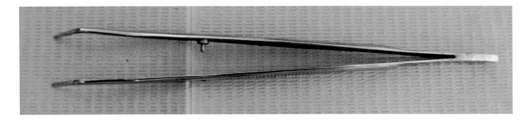

2. Cutting Instruments

There are three groups of cutting instruments: chisels, excavators, and carvers.

Chisels

Chisels are used for planning or cleaving unsupported enamel.

There are straight chisels, bi-angled chisels, and hatchet chisels for contouring class II preparations.

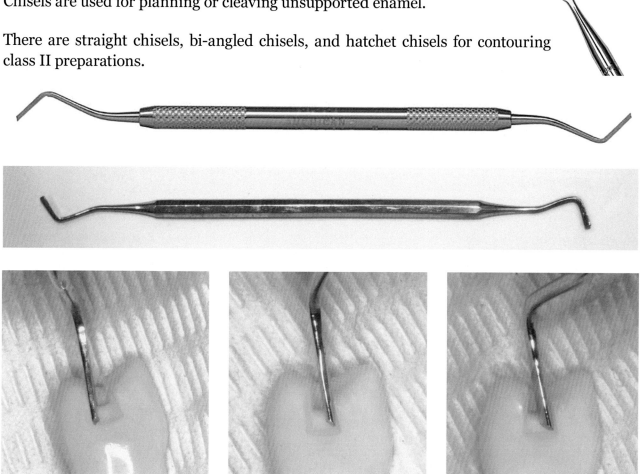

Directing the sharp blade of the hatchet with firm pressure can smooth and remove the unsupported enamel of the cavity.

Gingival margin trimmers are used to produce proper bevel on gingival enamel margins. They can also be used for bevelling the axio-pupal line angle

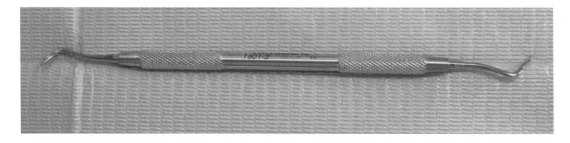

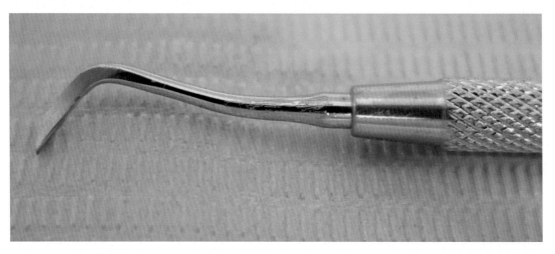

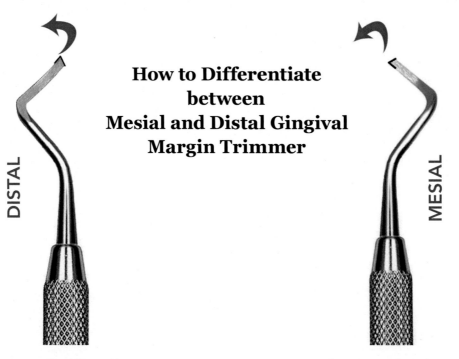

How to Differentiate between Mesial and Distal Gingival Margin Trimmer

DISTAL

MESIAL

Sharp end pointed away from the handle

Sharp end pointed towards the handle

Excavators

These tools remove the soft dentin and caries; secondary functions include removing temporary crowns and temporary cement in a temporary restoration and removing permanent crowns during try-in procedure.

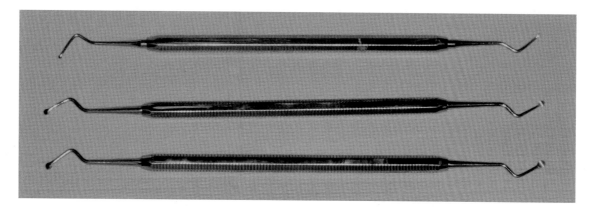

Carvers

These instruments are used to remove excess restorative materials and carve tooth anatomy in the restoration before the material hardens.

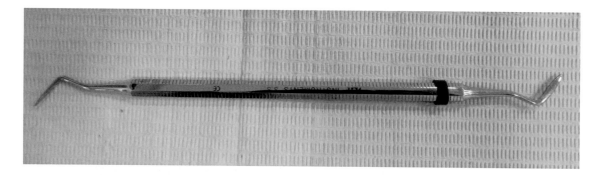

Hollenback carvers are used to shape the restoration.

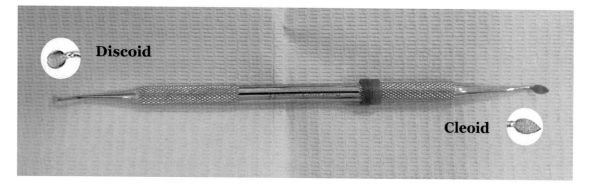

Discoid-cleoid carvers are used to shape amalgam restorations.

3. Noncutting Instruments

1. Amalgam Carrier

- carries and transfers amalgam to the prepared cavity
- aids in dispensing and placement of amalgam into the prepared cavity

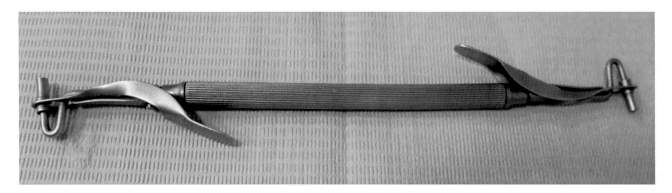

2. Condenser

- condense amalgam and other restorative materials in the prepared cavity

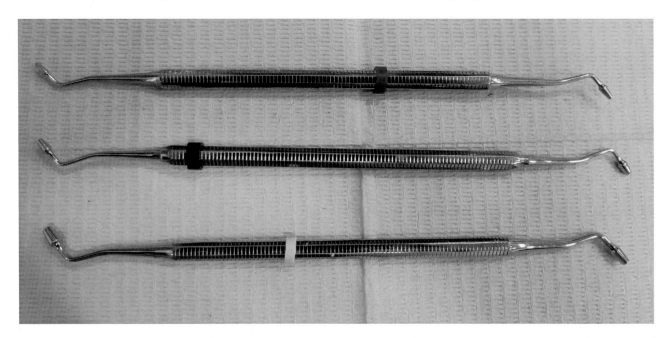

3. Burnishers (Ball, Ovoid, Anatomical)

- adapt amalgam to cavity margins
- aids initial shaping of restoration
- smoothening of the restoration surface
- shaping the metal matrix band

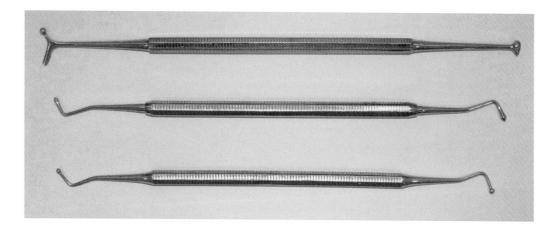

4. Plastic Instrument

- Used to transfer, place and shape cements and restorative materials.

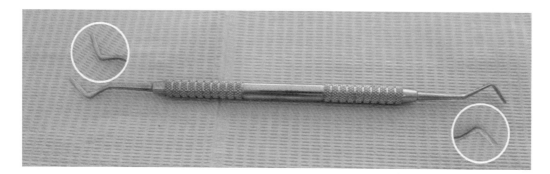

5. Cement Spatula

- used for mixing the different types of dental cements

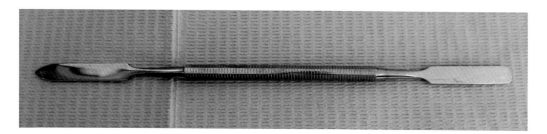

6. Metal Syringe

- used by dentists for injecting local anaesthetic

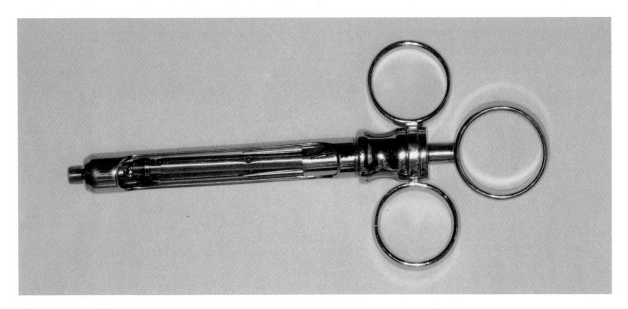

7. Dycal Applicator

- mall ball-pointed instrument that can be used to apply some dental liner and base material to the cavity pulp surfaces (e.g., Dycal or Vitrebond)

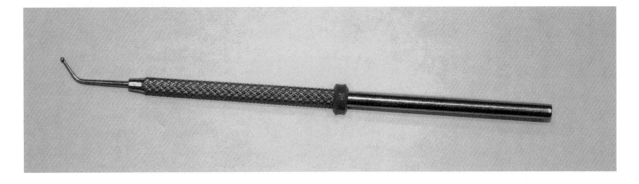

REFERENCES

1. Robinson, Debbie S., Bird, Doni L. (2017), *Modern Dental Assisting* 11th edition, Elsevier.
2. Heymann, Harald O., Swift, Edward J., and Ritter, Andre V. (2013), *Sturdevant's Art & Science of Operative Dentistry,* 6th edition, Elsevier.
3. Boyd, Linda Bartolomucci, (2017), *Dental Instruments: A Pocket Guide*, 6th Edition, Elsevier.
4. Gladwinand, M., and Bagby, M. (2018), *Clinical Aspects of Dental Materials: Theory, Practice, and Cases* 5th edition, Wolters Kluwer.
5. Garg, Nisha, Garg, Amit (2013), *Textbook of Operative Dentistry*, 2nd edition, Jaypee Brothers Medical Publishers.
6. Ireland, Robert (2010), *A Dictionary of Dentistry,* Oxford University Press.
7. Hilton, Thomas J., Ferracane, Jack L., Broome, James C. (2013), *Summitt's Fundamentals of Operative Dentistry: A Contemporary Approach*, 4th edition, Quintessence Publishing Co.

4

MATRICES

A matrix is a properly contoured temporary wall replacing the lost tooth structure due to caries, lesions, or other deformites.it is made of metal, plastic sheet, or other materials to maintain the restorative material within the cavity preparation.

Advantages

a. provides proximal and axial contour and contact
b. confines the restorative material within the cavity
c. prevents restoration excess

These are the most common matrices used in operative dentistry:

1. Universal Tofflemire Matrix Band and Retainer

- part of the matrix
- matrix band
- Tofflemire matrix retainer (also known as matrix band holder)

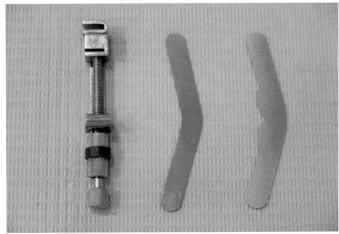

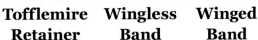

Tofflemire Retainer   **Wingless Band**   **Winged Band**

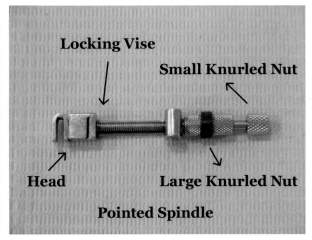

Tofflemire Matrix Application

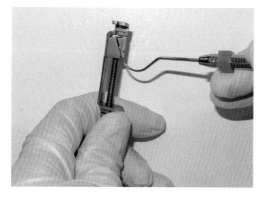
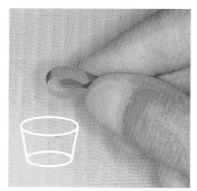
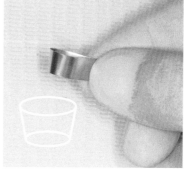

Make sure the head and the locking vise are in place and the bath for the band is clear.

Fold the matrix band to create a conical shape with two oval rings.

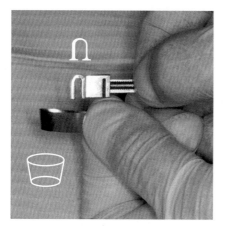
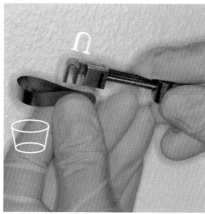
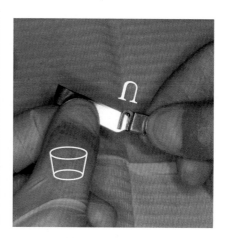

Fix the band on the retainer, directing the large circle of the conical band shape inside the U shape of the Tofflemire head.

As a rule, always direct the smaller ring and the U shape of the retainer towards the gingiva, no matter which tooth will be restored.

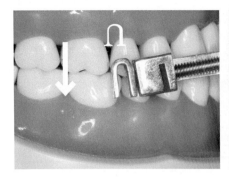
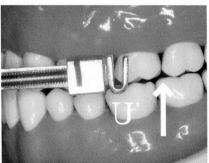
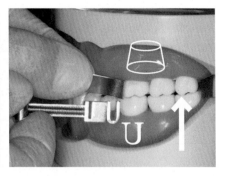

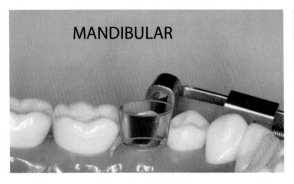
MANDIBULAR

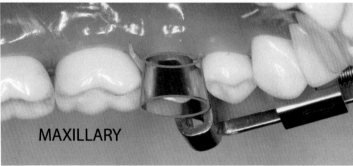
MAXILLARY

The smaller ring of the band and the U shape of the retainer head is directed to the gingiva.

Anterior Maxillary and Mandibular Teeth (Mesial and Distal)

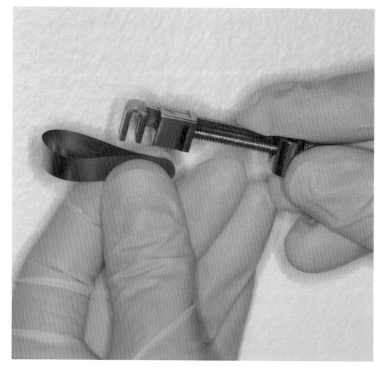 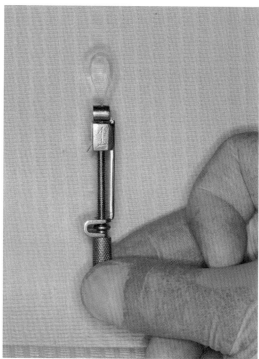

Making the band straight in the middle of the head of the retainer will suit the anterior maxillary and mandibular teeth.

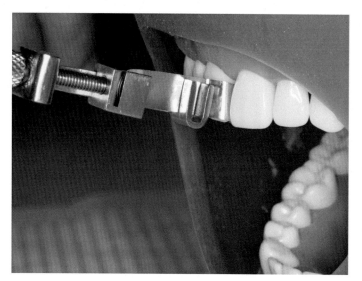 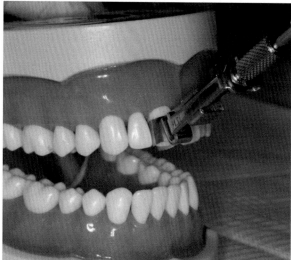

Posterior Mandibular Left and Maxillary Right Teeth Quadrants

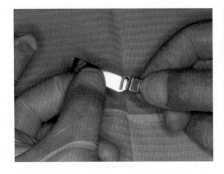 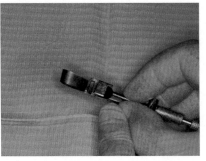 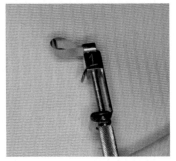

Directing the band to the left of the head of the retainer will suit the posterior lower left and upper right teeth quadrants in the same time.

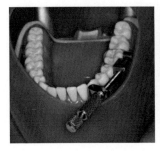 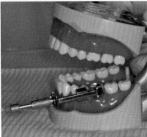 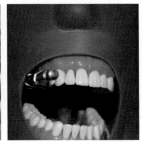 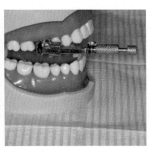

Posterior Mandibular Right and Maxillary Left Quadrant

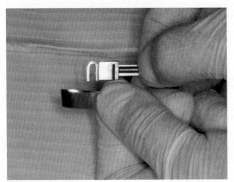 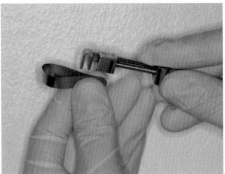 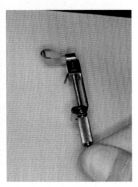

Directing the band to the right of the head of the retainer will suit posterior mandibular right and maxillary left quadrant at the same time.

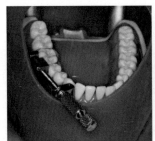 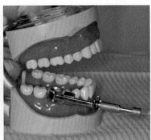 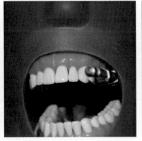 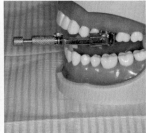

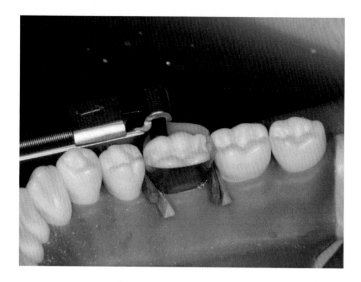

The band should be seated around the tooth such that:

The occlusal portion of the band extends 1–2 mm above the marginal ridge of the adjacent tooth and the cavosurface margin. This allows for proper condensation of the amalgam in the marginal ridge area.

The gingival portion of the band extends 0.5 mm below the gingival cavosurface margin and is supported with a wooden wedge.

2. Sectional Matrix System

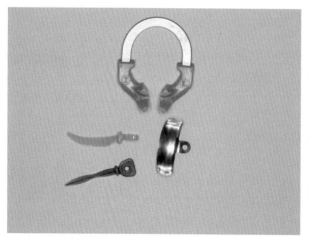
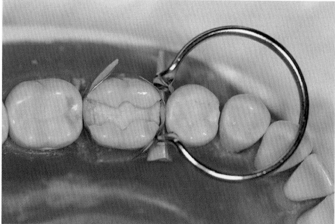

A. Sectional Matrix with Separating Rings

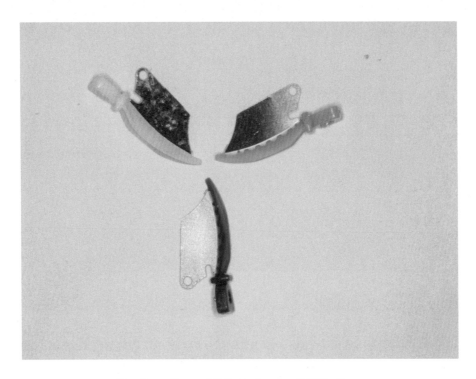

B. Sectional Matrix and Wedge

3. Automatrix

This technique allows matrix placement and retention without the need for bulky retainers, for ease of placement, better access, clear view of the operating field and greater patient comfort

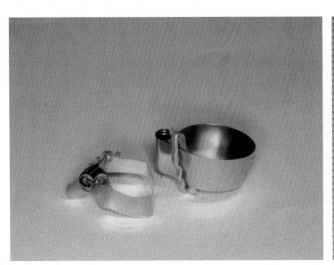
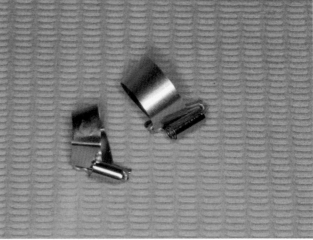

4. Clear Matrices

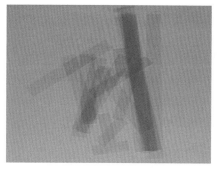

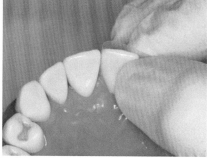

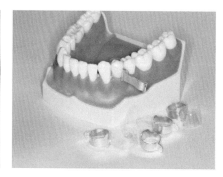

Polyester Strips **Mylar Strips** **Clear Plastic Crown Form**

5. Wedges

This is a small tapering triangular piece of wood, plastic, or other material to confine the matrix band to the proximal part of a cavity and prevent any restorative material leakage.

Advantages

- supports the band against the gingival margin to prevent leakage and overhang of the restorative material.
- protect gingival tissue
- separate the teeth to compensate for the thickness of the band

Most Common Wedges

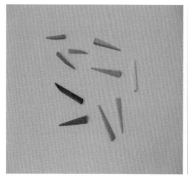

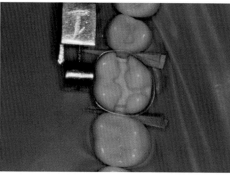

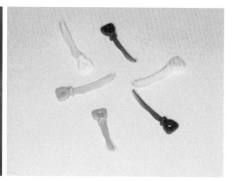

Wooden triangular and plastic wedges are most commonly used.

REFERENCES

1. Robinson, Debbie S., Bird, Doni L. (2017), *Modern Dental Assisting* 11th edition, Elsevier.
2. Heymann, Harald O., Swift, Edward J., and Ritter, Andre V. (2013), *Sturdevant's Art & Science of Operative Dentistry,* 6th edition, Elsevier.
3. Boyd, Linda Bartolomucci, (2017), *Dental Instruments: A Pocket Guide*, 6th Edition, Elsevier.
4. Gladwinand, M., and Bagby, M. (2018), *Clinical Aspects of Dental Materials: Theory, Practice, and Cases* 5th edition, Wolters Kluwer.
5. Garg, Nisha, Garg, Amit (2013), *Textbook of Operative Dentistry*, 2nd edition, Jaypee Brothers Medical Publishers.
6. Ireland, Robert (2010), *A Dictionary of Dentistry,* Oxford University Press
7. Hilton, Thomas J., Ferracane, Jack L., Broome, James C. (2013), *Summitt's Fundamentals of Operative Dentistry: A Contemporary Approach*, 4th edition, Quintessence Publishing Co.

5

INSTRUMENT HAND GRASPS AND RESTS

Manner of Holding the Instrument

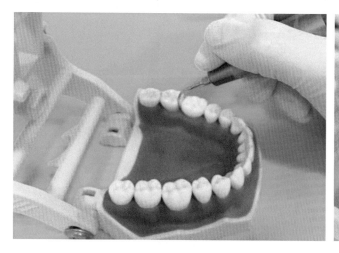

1. Pen grasp

2. Modified pen grasp

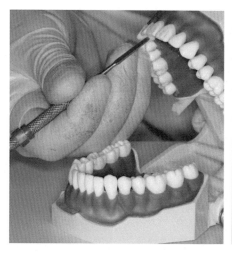

3. Inverted pen grasp

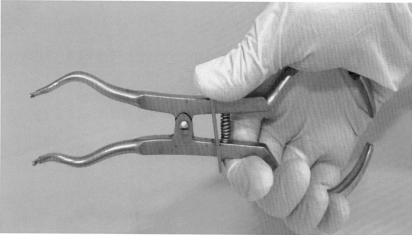

4. Palm and thumb grasp

Finger Rests and Support

1. Intra-Oral Finger Rest

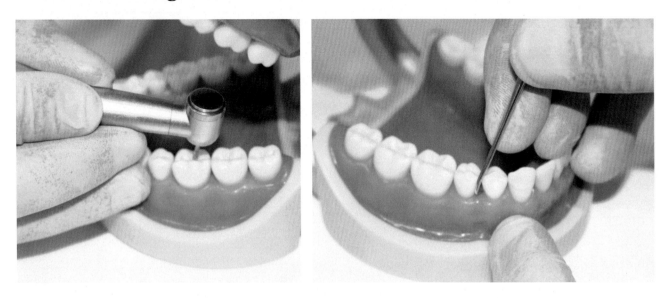

The conventional finger rest is just near or adjacent to the working tooth.

Cross Arch

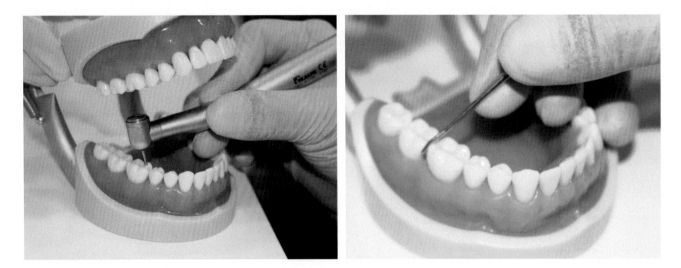

The finger rest is achieved from the tooth of the opposite site but of the same arch.

Opposite Arch

Finger on Finger

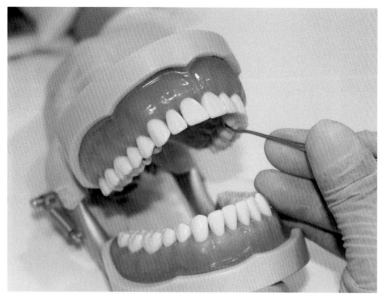

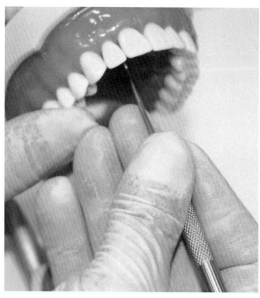

The finger rest is achieved from tooth of the opposite arch.

The rest is achieved from index finger or thumb of nonoperating hand.

Supporting High Speeds during Preparation

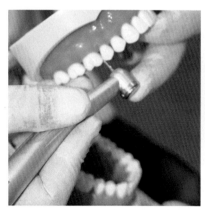 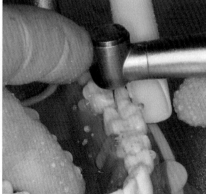 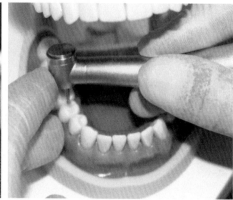

To avoid any unwanted injury to the tooth or soft tissue, it is recommended to support the handpiece head during operation as shown.

Indirect Vision Preparation

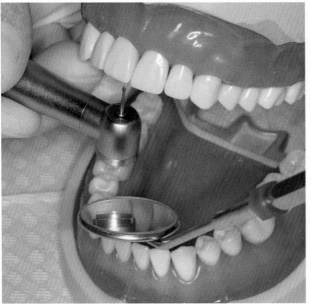 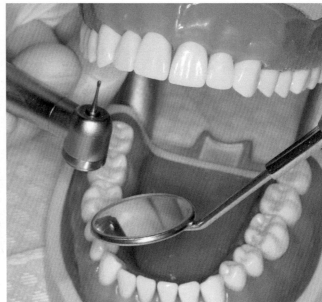

2. Extra-Oral Finger Rest

This is used mostly for maxillary posterior teeth.

Palm Up	**Palm Down**

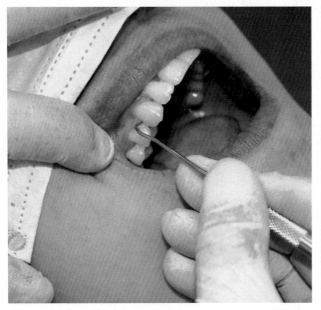 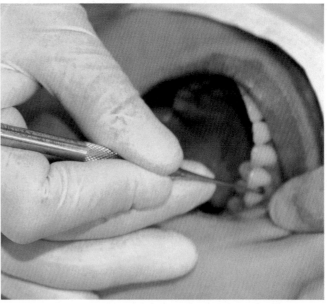

Rest is obtained by resting the back of the middle and fourth finger on the lateral of the mandible on the right side of the face.

Rest is obtained by resting the front surface of the middle and fourth fingers on the lateral of the mandible on the left side of the face.

REFERENCES

1. Robinson, Debbie S., Bird, Doni L. (2017), *Modern Dental Assisting* 11th edition, Elsevier.
2. Heymann, Harald O., Swift, Edward J., and Ritter, Andre V. (2013), *Sturdevant's Art & Science of Operative Dentistry,* 6th edition, Elsevier.
3. Gladwinand, M., and Bagby, M. (2018), *Clinical Aspects of Dental Materials: Theory, Practice, and Cases* 5th edition, Wolters Kluwer.
4. Garg, Nisha, Garg, Amit (2013), *Textbook of Operative Dentistry,* 2nd edition, Jaypee Brothers Medical Publishers.
5. Hilton, Thomas J., Ferracane, Jack L., Broome, James C. (2013), *Summitt's Fundamentals of Operative Dentistry: A Contemporary Approach*, 4th edition, Quintessence Publishing Co.

6

RUBBER DAM ISOLATION

A rubber dam (also known as dental dam) is a thin, rectangular sheet, usually latex rubber, used in dentistry to isolate the operative site (one or more teeth) from the rest of the mouth.

Uses of dental dams include the following:
- provide isolation for the operation area
- decrease saliva contamination
- reduce infection and cross contamination.
- prevent patient from swallowing any small particles
- protect soft tissues from sharp instruments and materials

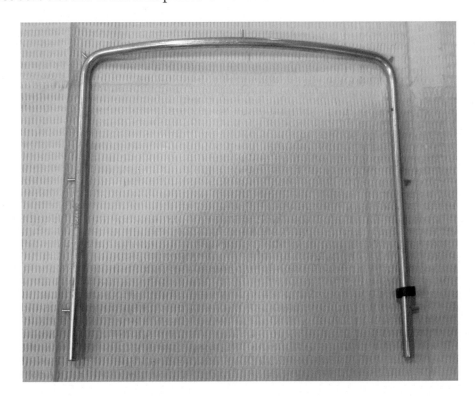

- **Rubber Dam Frame Holder (to keep dental dan away from the teeth)**

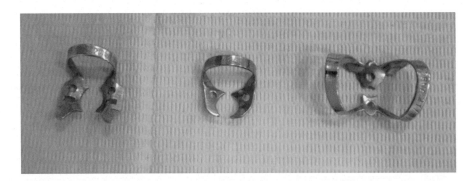

- **Rubber dam clamps (winged clamp-wingless clamp-cervical clamps)**

Winged Clamp - Wingless Clamp - Cervical Clamp

- **Rubber Dam Puncher (used to create holes in rubber dams)**

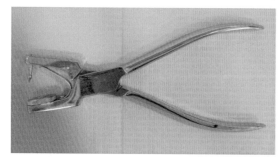 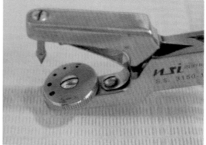

- **Rubber Dam Clamp Holder (used to hold the clamp or retainer)**

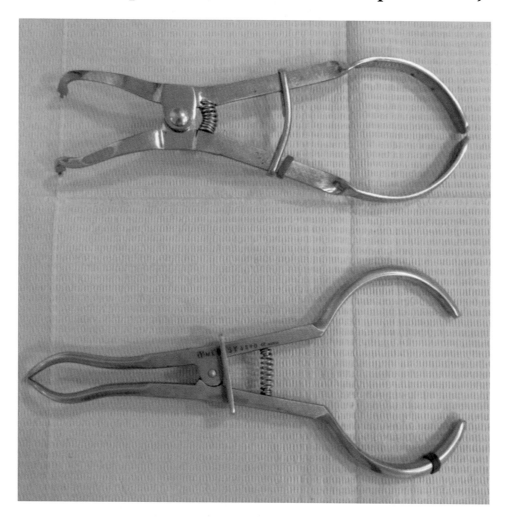

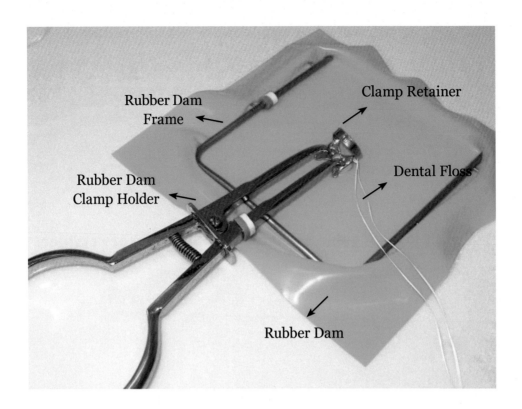

- Rubber Dam Frame
- Clamp Retainer
- Rubber Dam Clamp Holder
- Dental Floss
- Rubber Dam

Rubber Dam Application

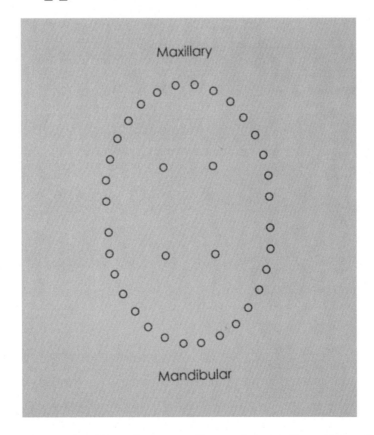

Maxillary

Mandibular

Use the commercial rubber dam template to locate the rubber dam holes.

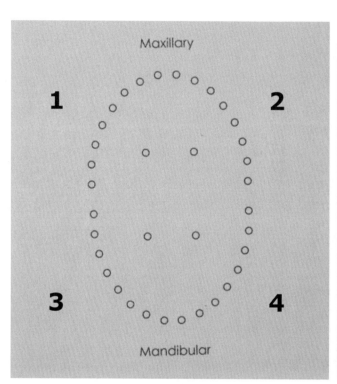

Divide the maxillary and mandibular teeth into four quadrants for more orientation.

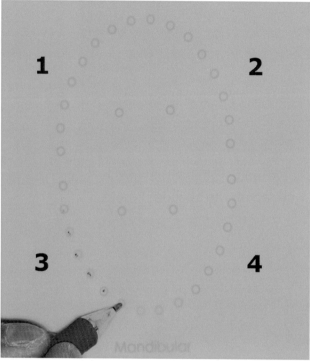

Mark the teeth to be isolated and the tooth to be the anchor. For minimal isolation, usually one to three teeth to be isolated anterior to the prepared tooth and one tooth distal.

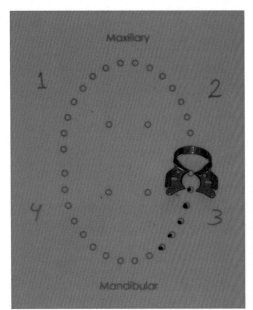

Estimate the position of the clamp on the anchored tooth.

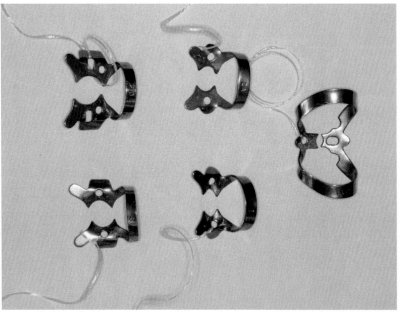

Ligate the clamp with dental floss for safety.

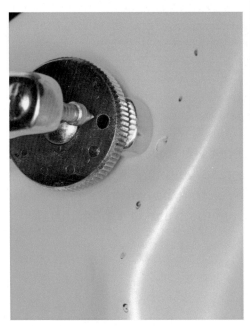

Punch the rubber dam exactly in the marked dots.

How to Place the Rubber Dam

1. With your assistant, place the rubber dam on the teeth to be isolated and then place the clamp over the anchored tooth.

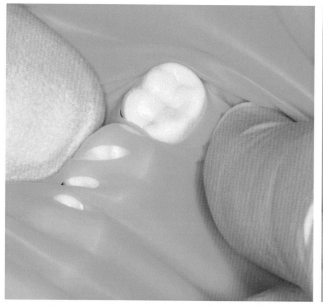
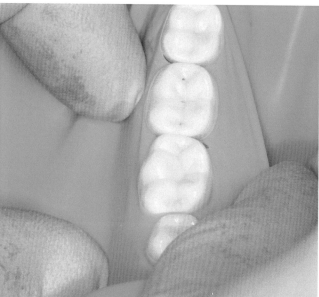

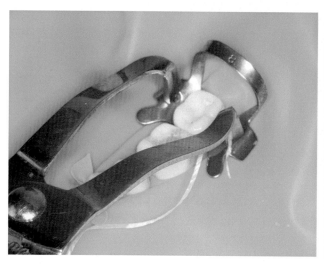
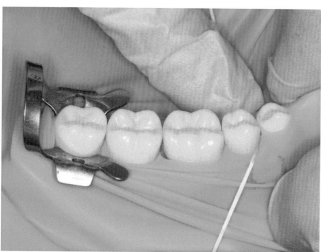

2. Place the clamp on the anchored tooth first and then start the other teeth to be isolated.

3. Use the dental floss to fix the septal section between the teeth.

Different Types of Operative Rubber Dam Isolation

1. Full arch (teeth isolation)

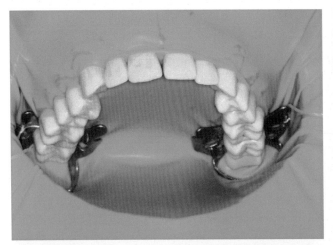 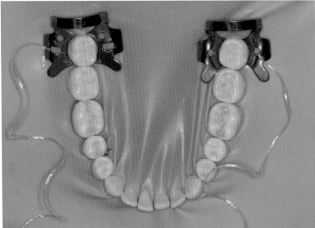

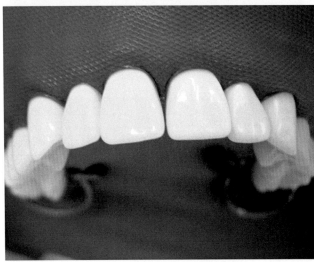 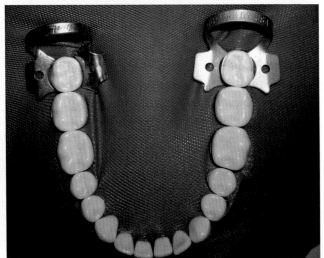

Upper Teeth   **Lower Teeth**

2. Full quadrant teeth isolation

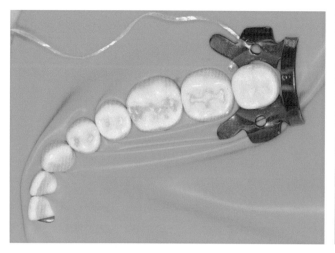 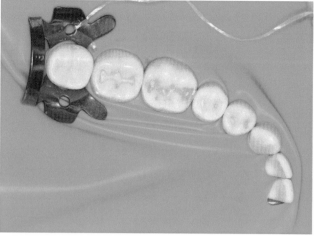

Right Side   **Left Side**

3. Anterior teeth isolation

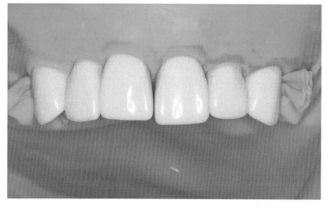 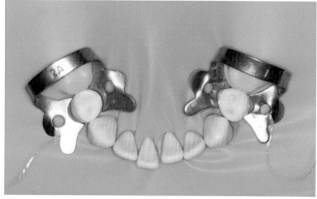

Fix anterior teeth with sectional rubber dam.   Fix anterior rubber dam with two clamps.

4. Two to three teeth isolation

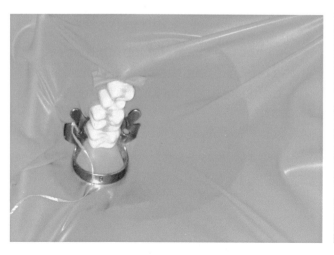 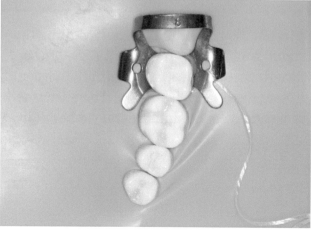

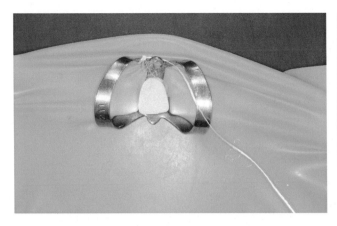
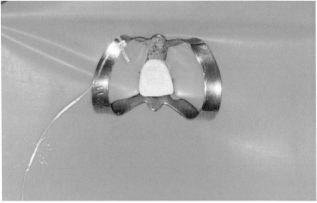

Removal of Rubber Dam

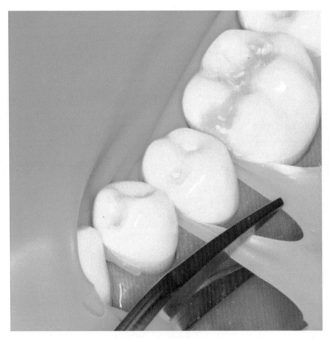
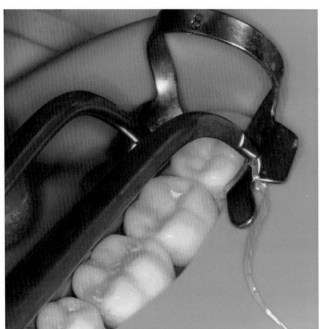

Stretch the rubber dam facially, pulling the septal rubber away from the gingival tissue. Place fingertip beneath the septum in order to protect the underlying tissue. Then use small scissors to cut the inter septal rubber dam.

Anchor the clamp forceps to remove the retainer and then release the dam from the anterior anchored tooth.

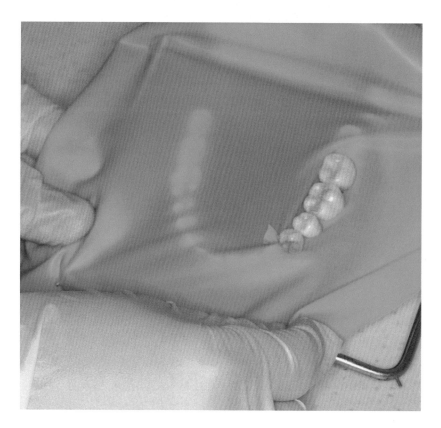

Remove the frame and the dam Simultaneously.

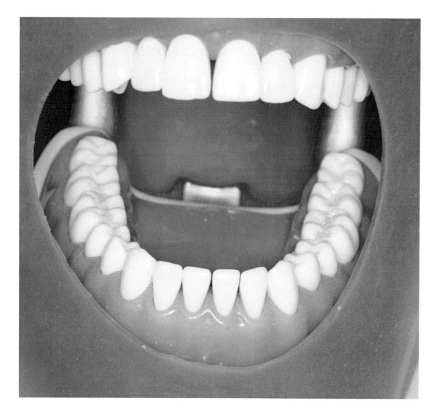

Check the interproximal areas with dental floss for any
fragments have been left between teeth.

REFERENCES

1. Robinson, Debbie S., Bird, Doni L. (2017), *Modern Dental Assisting* 11th edition, Elsevier.
2. Reid, James S., Callis, Paul D., Patterson, Colin J. W. (1991), *Rubber Dam in Clinical Practice*, Quintessence Publishing.
3. Boyd, Linda Bartolomucci, (2017), *Dental Instruments: A Pocket Guide*, 6th Edition, Elsevier.
4. Gladwinand, M., and Bagby, M. (2018), *Clinical Aspects of Dental Materials: Theory, Practice, and Cases* 5th edition, Wolters Kluwer.
5. Hilton, Thomas J., Ferracane, Jack L., Broome, James C. (2013), *Summitt's Fundamentals of Operative Dentistry: A Contemporary Approach*, 4th edition, Quintessence Publishing Co.

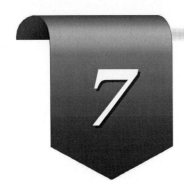

7

ANATOMICAL LANDMARKS

Tooth Anatomy Related to Operative Dentistry

Enamel

This is the hard tissue that covers the crown portion of the tooth (hardest substance in the body).

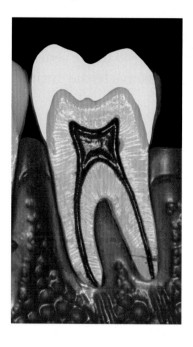

Importance

1. Caries lesion start from enamel and can spread to dentin.
2. Simple cavity preparation could be preventive resin restoration or fissure sealant when caries affect only enamel tissue of the tooth.

Dentin

This is the material forming the main inner portion of the tooth structure and surrounding the pulp.

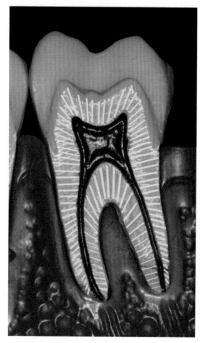

Importance

1. If caries reach the dentin, it spreads fast.
2. Dentin is not as hard as enamel.
3. Simple to moderate or complicated cavity preparation would be the result of dentin caries severity.

Cementum

This is the substance covering the root surface of the tooth.

Importance

1. Caries affect the cementum if the gingival tissue is receded as a consequence of periodontal disease or if the cervical caries spread to the cementum through coronal dentin.
2. Avoid injury the pulp and the sensitive tissue during cavity preparation in cementum.

Pulp

The pulp is the vital tissues of the tooth consisting of nerves, blood vessels, and connective tissue.

Importance

1. In operative dentistry, give great attention to protect the pulp from restoration material irritation by using specific liner and base material suitable for the restorative material used.
2. Many preparation techniques for cavity preparation give great attention to protect the pulp and avoid injuring it.

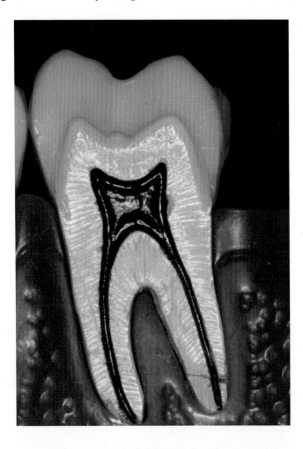
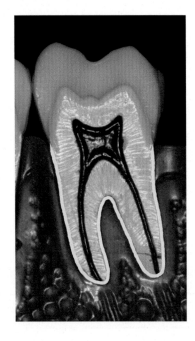

Smooth Surface Terminology

- **Mesial.** The surfaces of the tooth directed towards the central line (midline) of the dental arch, as opposed to distal.
- **Distal.** The surfaces of the tooth directed away from the central line (midline) of the dental arch.
- **Facial.** Teeth surfaces opposed and in contact with the cheek tissue in both maxillary and mandibular teeth.
- **Labial.** This surface of an anterior tooth faces towards the lips in both maxillary and mandibular teeth.
- **Lingual.** The surfaces of a tooth facing towards the tongue in the mandibular teeth.
- **Palatal.** Surfaces of the teeth facing the palate in the maxillary teeth (palate is the roof of the mouth).
- **Occlusal surface.** The surfaces of premolars and molars that come in contact with those in opposite jaws during the act of closure are called occlusal surfaces.
- **Incisal surface.** The surfaces of incisors and canines that come in contact with those in the opposite jaws during the act of closure are called incisal surfaces
- **Gingival or cervical.** Portion of the teeth near to the gingiva or gum line.
- **Proximal.** The mesial or distal surface of a tooth or the portion of a cavity that is near to the adjacent tooth.

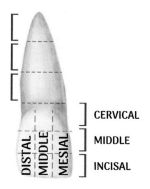

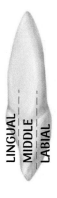

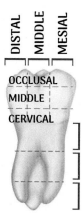

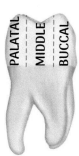

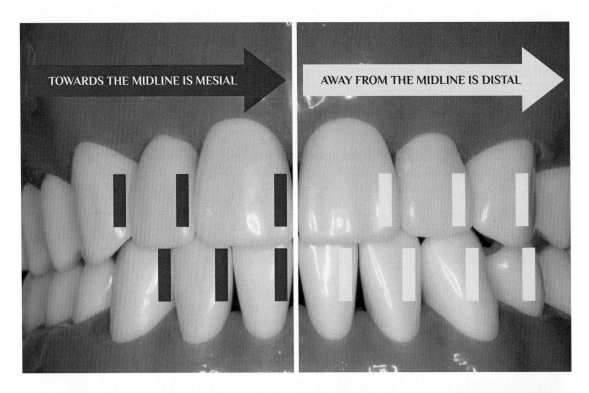

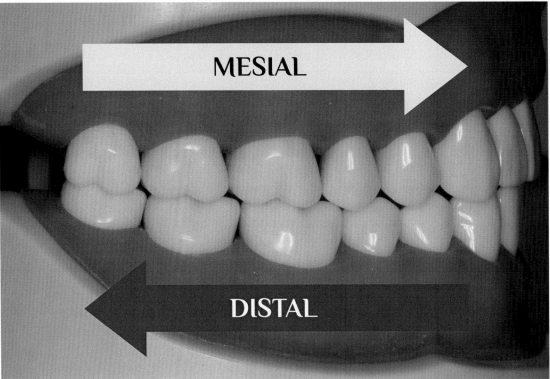

Importance

More specifications for the types and severity of the caries lesions and their diagnosis and operative dental treatment.

Pits and Fissures

Pit

Pinpoint depression located in the pinpoint junction of development grooves or fissures or sharp pinpoint depression on the surface of enamel.

Importance

1. Most common site for caries
2. Usually need fissure sealant for caries prevention or treatment.

Fissure

This is an incomplete joining along the developmental groove during the union of the two lobes.

Importance

1. Commonly affected by caries lesion.
2. Fissure restoration should include unaffected fissures by caries for prevention because of the possibility of future caries.

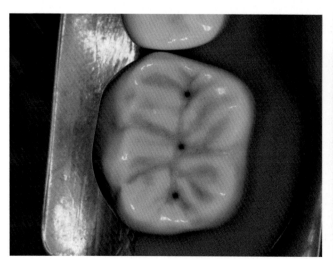
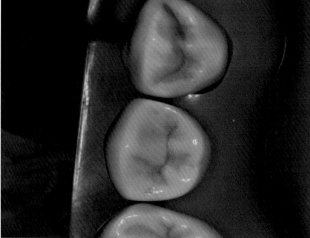

Fossa

Round or irregular depression found on the lingual surface of most anterior teeth and on occlusal surface of posterior teeth.

The depression on the lingual surface of an anterior tooth bordered by the incisal edge, the cingulum, and the marginal ridges. Sometimes referred to as the lingual concavity.

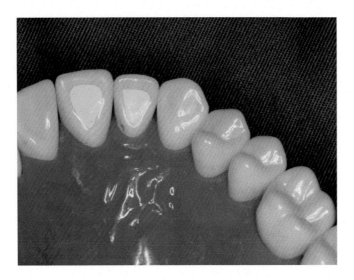

Palatal or Lingual Fossa

Triangular Fossa in Posterior Teeth

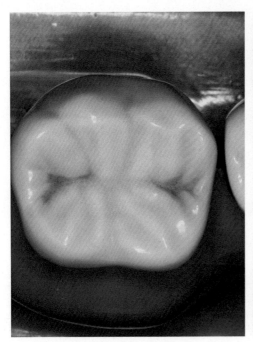

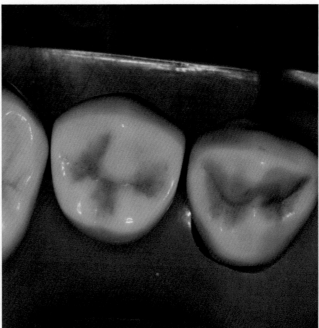

Triangular Fossa　　　　　　　**Central Fossa**

Cingulum

Bulge or elevation located on the lingual cervical third of anterior teeth (lingual lobe of anterior teeth).

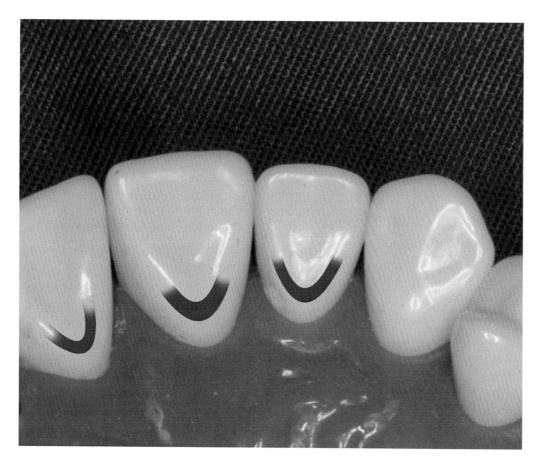

Importance

Lingual pit caries sometimes occur near the cingulum.

Lobe

This is one of the primary sections of formation in development of a crown.

Cusps and Mamelons are representative of lobes.

Cusp

This is a peak or elevation of a tooth located on the occlusal surface of molars and premolars and on the incisal edges of canines.

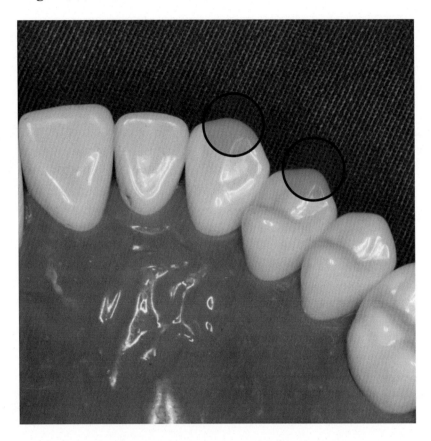

Cuspal tips are pointed or rounded projections on the crown of the tooth.

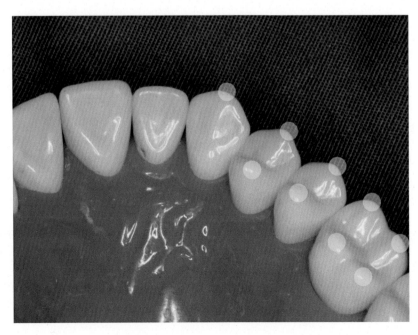

Cusps of Carabelli

A Fifth Cusp Found on the Lingual Surface of Some Max First Molars

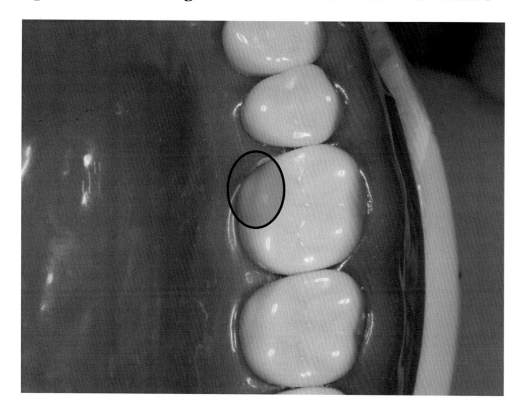

Mamelons

Three rounded protuberances found on incisal ridges of newly erupted incisor.

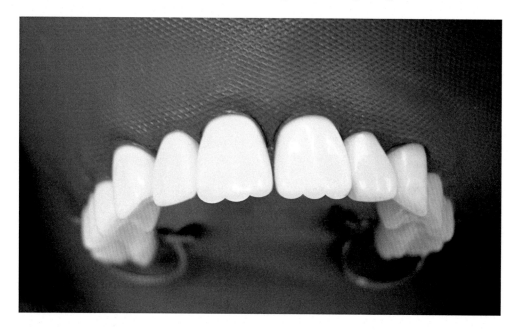

Cusp incline/slope

is the sloping area found between two cusp ridges.

Cusp ridges

Each cusp has four cusp ridges extending in different directions (mesial, distal, facial, and lingual) from the cusp tip.

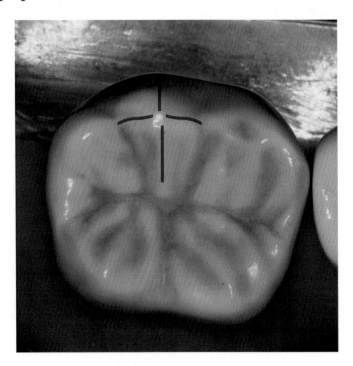

Ridges

This linear elevation (slope) on the surface of a tooth gets its name from its location.

Triangular ridges are cusp ridges that extend towards the central portion of occlusal surface.

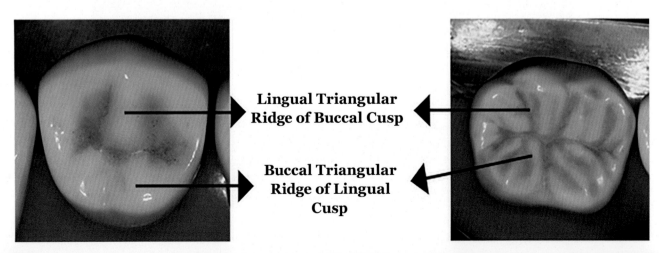

Lingual Triangular Ridge of Buccal Cusp

Buccal Triangular Ridge of Lingual Cusp

Transverse ridges

form when a buccal and lingual triangular ridge joint. Mostly found in the mandibular premolars.

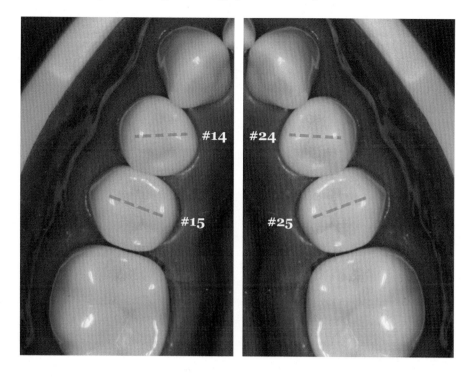

Oblique ridges

cross the occlusal surfaces of maxillary molars and formed by the union of the triangular ridge of the distobuccal cusp and the distal cusp ridge of the mesiolingual cusp.

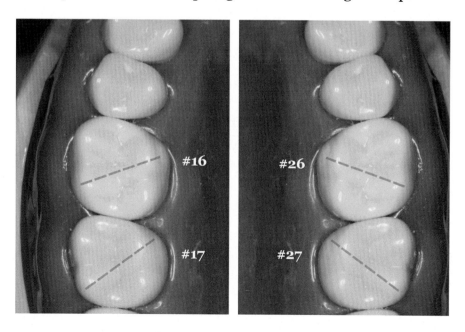

Marginal ridges

are rounded borders of enamel that form the mesial and distal margins of the occlusal surfaces of premolars and molars and the mesial and distal margins of the lingual surfaces of the incisors and canines.

Importance

1. All ridges and cusps help for proper mastication.
2. Cavities include those ridges in cavity preparation, should be regained in the new restoration.

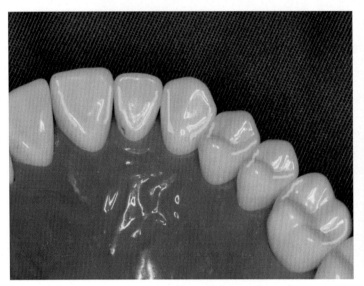 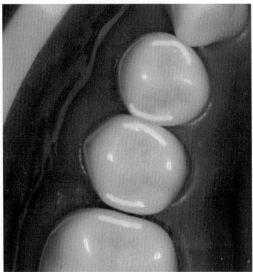

Contact

This is the area where teeth touch each other usually in mesial and distal surface area.

The contact area between teeth create embrasures in all directions.

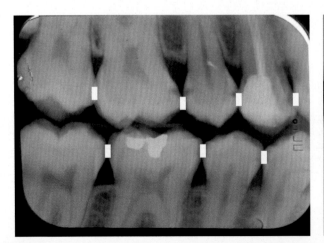 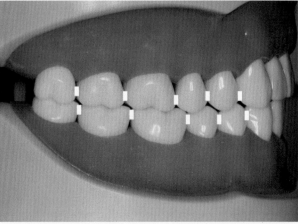

Importance

1. Proximal caries are formed in the contact area and beneath the contact area cervically
2. During cavity preparation for amalgam restoration, proximal contact should be broken for clearance of explorer tip width.
3. During cavity preparation for composite restoration, preserve the proximal contact and should not be broken for clearance, unless it's infected with caries.
4. Regain the contact after restoring proximal cavity restoration to have the same tight contact before preparation or before caries destruction.

Embrasures

Embrasures are v-shaped spaces around the proximal contacts existing between two adjacent teeth.

Embrasure spaces provide an escape route for food to pass during chewing.

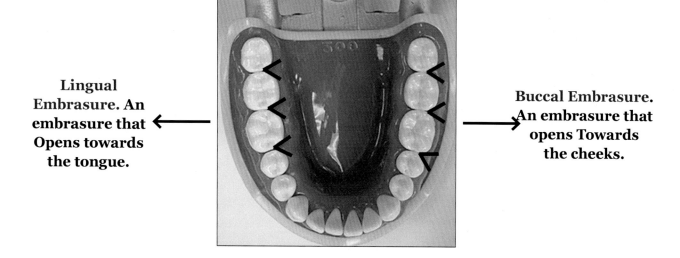

Lingual Embrasure. An embrasure that Opens towards the tongue.

Buccal Embrasure. An embrasure that opens Towards the cheeks.

Incisal Embrasures. An embrasure between the curved proximal surfaces of adjacent anterior teeth, incisal to the proximal contact.

Gingival Embrasures. An embrasure opening between the curved proximal surfaces of adjacent teeth, gingival to the proximal contact.

Occlusal Embrasures. An embrasure that opens towards the occlusal surface or plane.

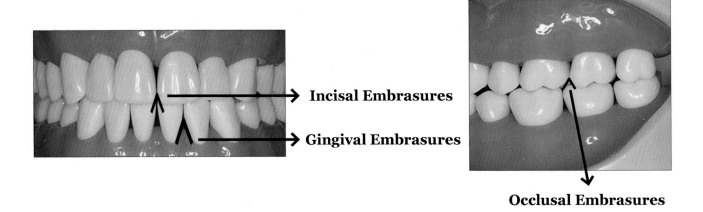

Incisal Embrasures

Gingival Embrasures

Occlusal Embrasures

Importance

1. Embrasure spaces provide an escape route for food to pass during chewing.
2. During cavity restoring, it is very important to restore all embrasures included in the cavity to their normal and actual form.

Groove

A linear depression on the surface of a tooth.

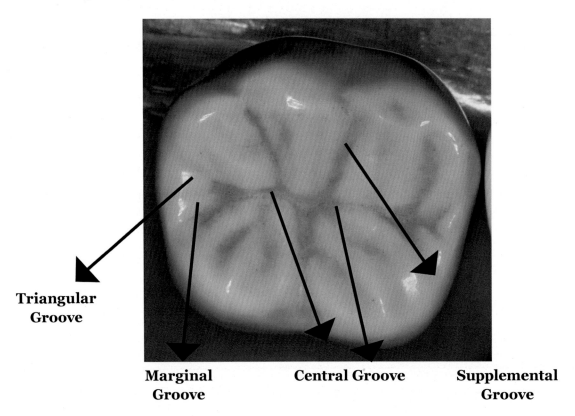

Triangular Groove

Marginal Groove

Central Groove

Supplemental Groove

Developmental Groove

This is a groove formed by the union of two lobes during the development of a crown; for example, buccal and lingual grooves.

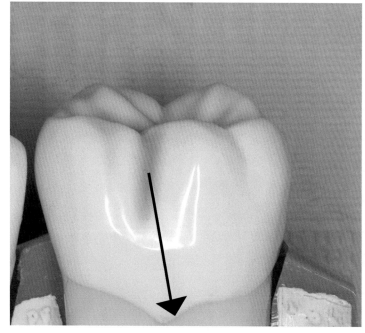

Buccal Groove

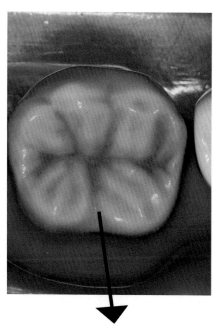

Lingual Groove

The central groove is the line depression dividing the occlusal surface of molars and premolars into two halves (buccal and lingual).

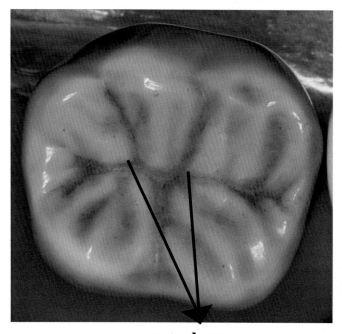

central grooves

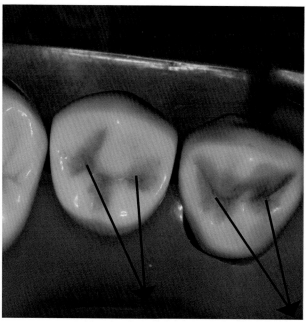

central grooves   central grooves

Supplemental groove

A shallow linear depression that is less distant than in a developmental groove. It gives the occlusal surface a wrinkled appearance.

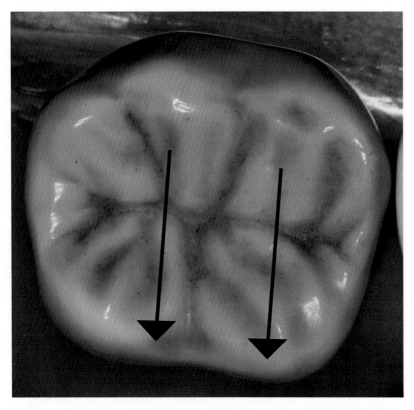

Supplemental groove

Importance

Grooves are more prone to caries like pits and fissures; restoration should have grooves but less deep than natural to prevent accumulation of food.

REFERENCES

1. Robinson, Debbie S., Bird, Doni L. (2017), *Modern Dental Assisting* 11th edition, Elsevier.
2. Heymann, Harald O., Swift, Edward J., and Ritter, Andre V. (2013), *Sturdevant's Art & Science of Operative Dentistry*, 6th edition, Elsevier.
3. Woelfel, Julian B., Scheid, Rickne C. (2011), *Woelfel's Dental Anatomy: Its Relevance to Dentistry*, 8th edition, Lippincott Williams & Wilkins.
4. Garg, Nisha, Garg, Amit (2013), *Textbook of Operative Dentistry*, 2nd edition, Jaypee Brothers Medical Publishers.
5. Nelson, Stanley J. (2015), *Wheeler's Dental Anatomy*, 10th edition, Elsevier.
6. Hilton, Thomas J., Ferracane, Jack L., Broome, James C. (2013), *Summitt's Fundamentals of Operative Dentistry: A Contemporary Approach*, 4th edition, Quintessence Publishing Co.

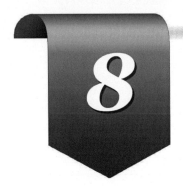

TOOTH CAVITY TERMINOLOGY

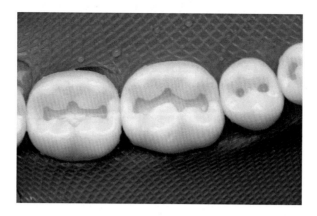

Cavity. Damaged areas in the tooth structure due to the carious lesion (both in enamel and dentin).

Cavity preparation. Mechanical alteration of a tooth structure to receive a restorative material to return the tooth to proper anatomical function and aesthetics form.

Simple tooth preparation. Cavity preparation that involves only one surface of a tooth (e.g., occlusal cavity preparation).

Compound tooth preparation. Cavity preparation that involves two surfaces of the tooth (e.g., class II Mesio-occlusal cavity preparation).

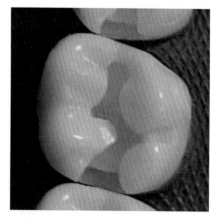

Complex tooth preparation. Cavity preparation that involves three or more surfaces of the tooth (e.g., class II Mesio-Occluso-distal cavity preparation).

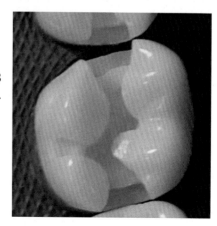

Internal wall. Cavity walls that is inside the tooth and does not extend to external tooth

Surface.

1. Axial wall. Internal wall that is parallel with the long axis of the tooth.
2. Pulpal wall. Internal wall that is perpendicular to the long axis of the tooth and occlusal of pulp.

External wall. Prepared surface that extends to the external surface of the tooth (e.g., facial, mesial, distal, lingual, and gingival walls)

Floor or Seat. Prepared wall that is relatively flat and perpendicular to the occlusal forces that are directed along the long axis of the tooth (e.g., pulpal and gingival seat).

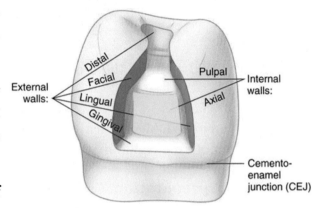

Angles in a cavity preparation. Junction of the two or more surfaces of a cavity preparation.

Line angle. Junction between two walls in the cavity preparation along a definite line.

Point angle. Junction of the three walls in a cavity preparation at a point.

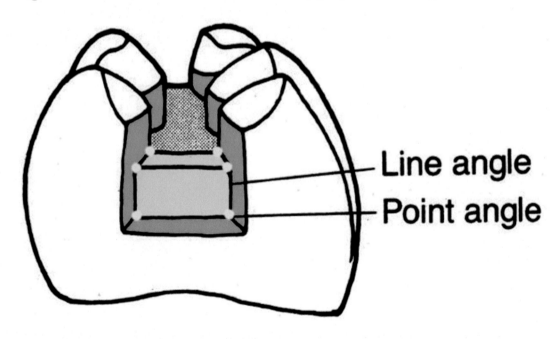

- Disto Facio Pulpal Angle (DFP)
- Facio Pulpal Angle (FP)
- Mesio Facio Pulpal Angle (MFP)

- Disto Facial Angle (DF)
- Disto Pupal Angle (DP)
- Disto Lingual Angle (DL)

- Disto Linguo Pulpal Angle (DLP)
- Linguo Pulpal Angle (LP)
- Mesiolingual Pulpal Angle (MLP)

- Mesio Facial Angle (MF)
- Mesio Pulpal Angle (MP)
- Mesiolingual Angle (ML)

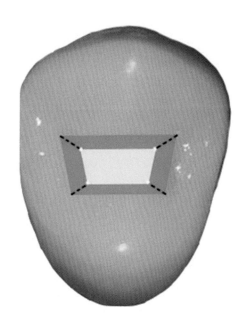

Cavosurface margin. The actual junction of the prepared wall and the external tooth surface.

Cavosurface angle. Angle of the tooth structure formed by the junction of a prepared wall and the external tooth surface.

Cavosurface Margin

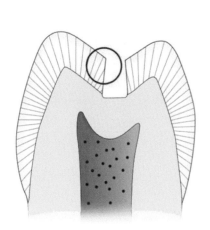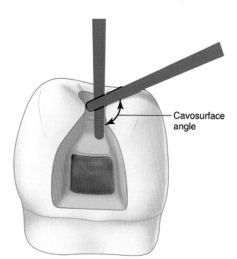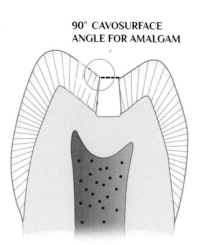

Cavosurface angle

90° CAVOSURFACE ANGLE FOR AMALGAM

REFERENCES

1. Banerjee, Avijit, Watson, Timothy F. (2015), *Pickard's Guide to Minimally Invasive Operative Dentistry*, 10th edition, Oxford Medical Publication.
2. Heymann, Harald O., Swift, Edward J., and Ritter, Andre V. (2013), *Sturdevant's Art & Science of Operative Dentistry,* 6th edition, Elsevier.
3. Garg, Nisha, Garg, Amit (2013), *Textbook of Operative Dentistry*, 2nd edition, Jaypee Brothers Medical Publishers.
4. Hilton, Thomas J., Ferracane, Jack L., Broome, James C. (2013), *Summitt's Fundamentals of Operative Dentistry: A Contemporary Approach*, 4th edition, Quintessence Publishing Co.

9

CLASSIFICATION OF CARIES LESIONS

G. V. Black's system for classifying caries lesions is used by dentists around the world. The principles for Black's classification and disease management system are more than a hundred years old, but they still hold true.

Class I Lesions

All pit-and-fissure caries are Class I, and they involve the following three location groups:

- **the occlusal surfaces of molars and premolars**
- **the occlusal two-thirds of the buccal and lingual surfaces of molars**
- **the lingual surfaces of anterior teeth**

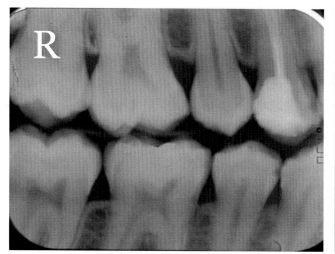
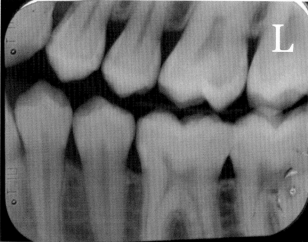
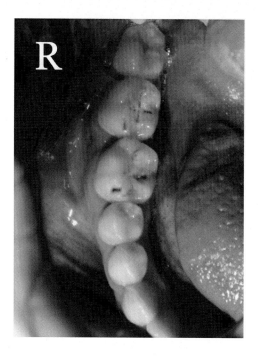
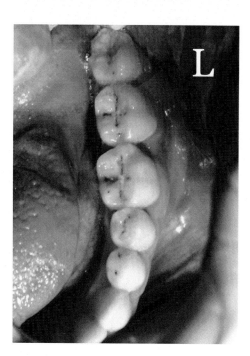

Class II Lesions

These involve the proximal surfaces (mesial and distal) of posterior teeth, with access established from the occlusal tooth surface.

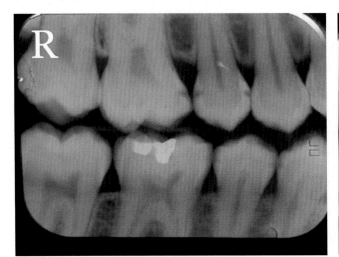
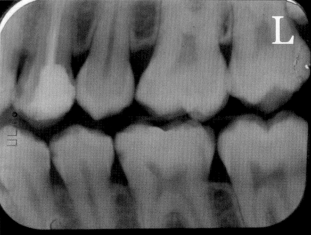

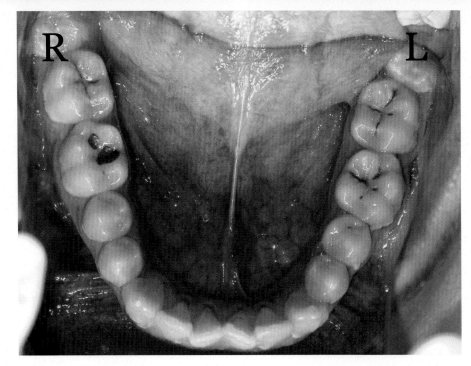

Class III Lesions

These involve the proximal surfaces of the anterior teeth that may or may not involve the lingual extension but do not involve the incisal line angle.

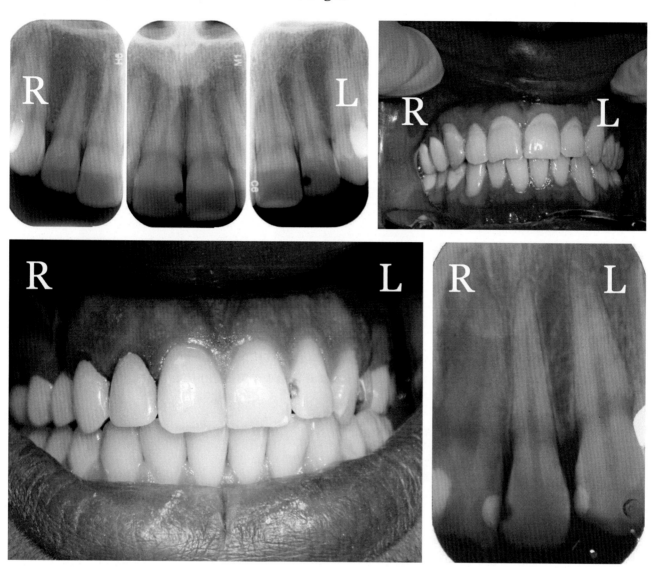

Class IV Lesions

Caries that involved all proximal surfaces of anterior teeth, also affects the incisal line angle.

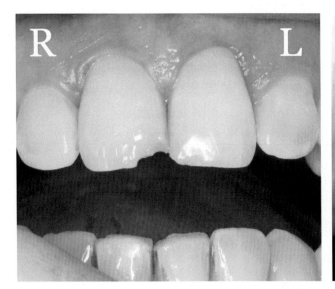 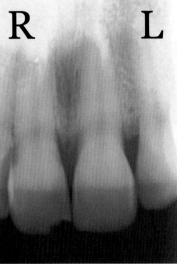

Class V Lesions

These involve the cervical third of all teeth, including the proximal surface of posterior teeth where the marginal ridge is not included in the cavity preparation (this does not involve pit or fissure areas).

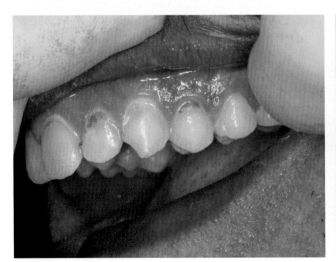 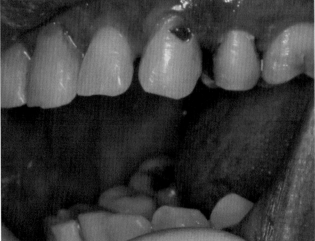

Class VI Lesions

Caries affecting the incisal edges of all anterior teeth and the cusp tips of all posterior teeth.

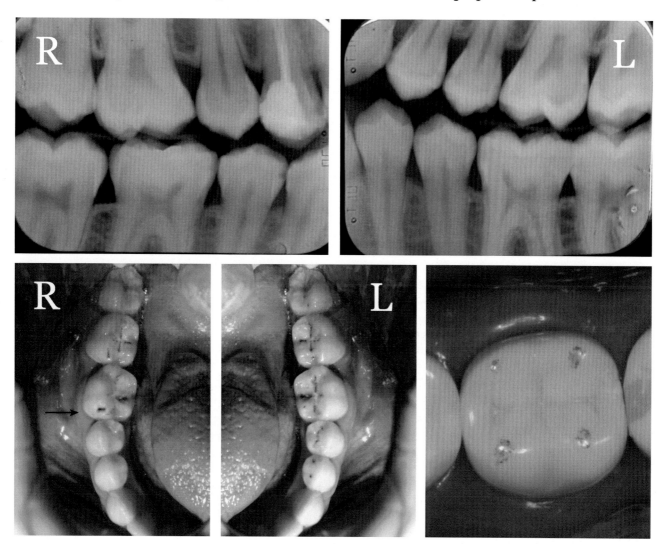

REFERENCES

1. Banerjee, Avijit, Watson, Timothy F. (2015), *Pickard's Guide to Minimally Invasive Operative Dentistry*, 10th edition, Oxford Medical Publication.
2. Black, G.V. (1908), *Operative Dentistry*, Vol. 1.
3. Heymann, Harald O., Swift, Edward J., and Ritter, Andre V. (2013), *Sturdevant's Art & Science of Operative Dentistry*, 6th edition, Elsevier.
4. Garg, Nisha, Garg, Amit (2013), *Textbook of Operative Dentistry*, 2nd edition, Jaypee Brothers Medical Publishers.
5. Hilton, Thomas J., Ferracane, Jack L., Broome, James C. (2013), *Summitt's Fundamentals of Operative Dentistry: A Contemporary Approach*, 4th edition, Quintessence Publishing Co.

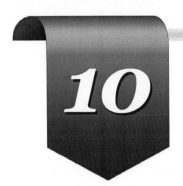

10

STEPS OF CAVITY PREPARATION

1. Initial Stage of Tooth Preparation

A. Outline Form (defined as shape of completed cavity including all caries extension)
B. Primary Resistance Form
C. Primary Retention Form

Parallelism or slight occlusal convergence 6–8° of two or more opposing, external walls.

D. Convenience Form

Adequate width and depth of outline form to allow operative instrumentation. Ideal width is one-third to one-quarter of the intercuspal distance.

2. Final Stage of Tooth Preparation

A. Removal of the Remaining Carious Dentin
B. Pulp Protection
C. Obtaining Secondary Resistance and Retention Form
D. Finishing of Enamel Wall and Margins
E. Cleaning and Disinfecting

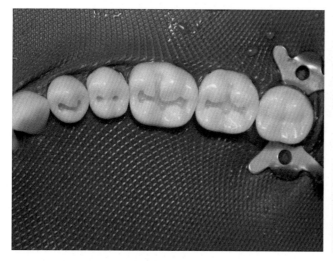 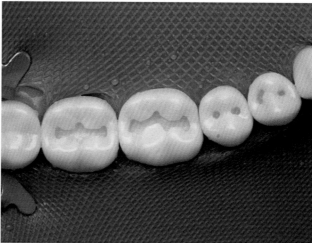

Class I Cavity Preparations and Their Corresponding Restorations

Cavity Preparation for Class I Amalgam Restoration

For easy cavity preparation, you could draw the caries lesion on an ivory tooth using sharp pensile in the deepest fossa and fissures to create the outline of the caries extension and for the cavity outline later.

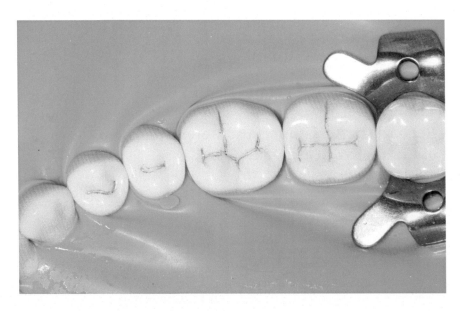

#36 and #37 Occlusal Caries with Buccal Extension
#34 and #35 Occlusal Caries

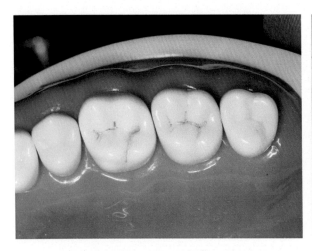

#16 Occlusal Caries (Not Including the Oblique Ridge)
#17 Occlusal Caries

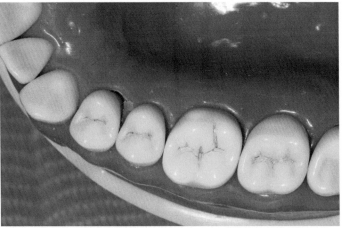

#24, #25, and #27 Occlusal Caries
#26 Occlusal Caries Crossing the Oblique Ridge with Palatal Extension

How Cavity Preparation Is Divided

1. Initial Stage of Tooth Preparation

A. Outline Form (Defined as Shape of Completed Cavity, Including All Caries Extension)

B. Primary Resistance Form
- Flat pulpal floor
- Minimal extension
- Initial depth (1–1.5 mm)

C. Primary Retention Form
- Parallelism or slight occlusal convergence (6–8°) of two or more opposing, external walls

D. Convenience Form
- Adequate width and depth of outline form to allow operative instrumentation.
- Ideal width is one-third to one-quarter of the intercuspal distance

Bur Orientation

It is important during dental treatments to orient the bur to be with the long axis of the tooth crown and perpendicular to the occlusal surface.

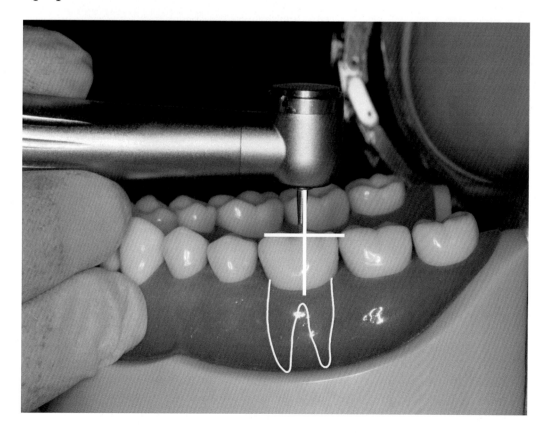

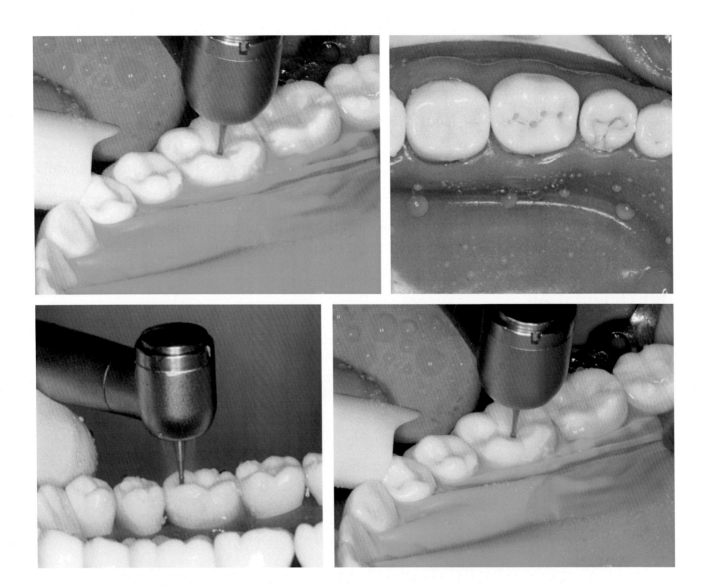

For beginners, create small drilling guiding holes, resampling the
cavity outline using small round burs; the dots can be created in the
deepest fossa and fissures to create the outline of the cavity.

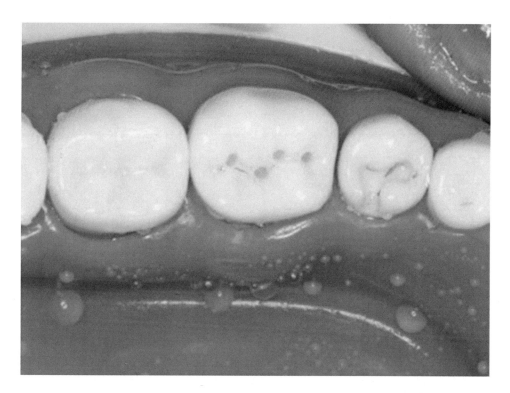

Then connect the dots with the same depth and width of the bur to create the initial outline form.

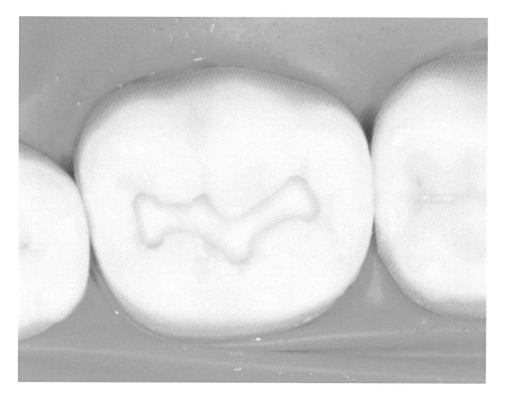

Initial Tooth Cavity Preparation

2. Final Stage of Tooth Preparation

A. Remove the Remaining Carious Dentin
B. Protect the Pulp
C. Obtain Secondary Resistance and Retention Form
D. Finish Enamel Wall and Margins
E. Clean and Disinfect

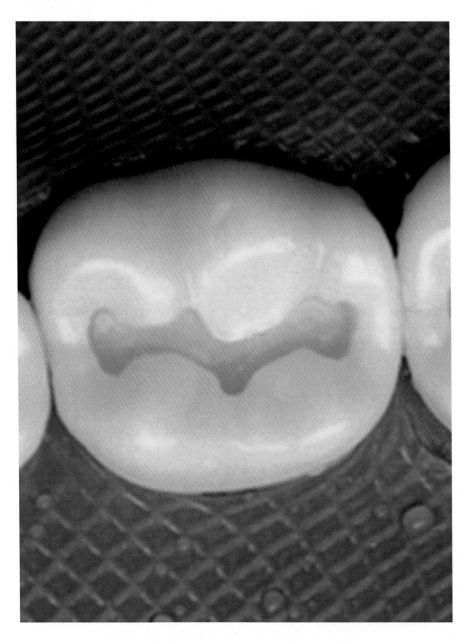

Final Class I Cavity Preparation

Steps for Amalgam Restoration in Class I Cavity Preparation

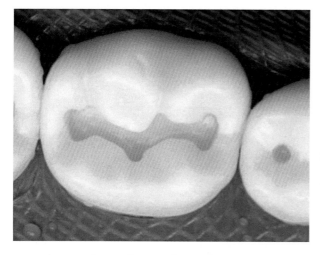

1. Dry the cavity prior to amalgam restoration.

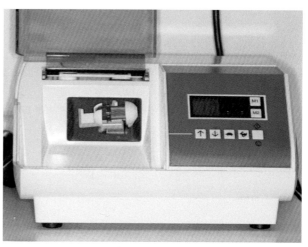

2. Activate the amalgam using amalgamator as per manufacturer instructions.

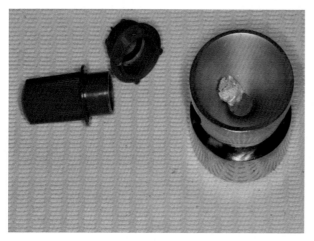

3. Release the amalgam in the amalgam well.

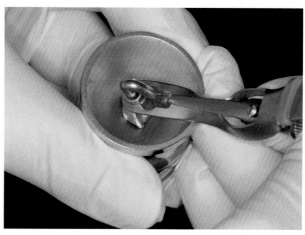

4. Load the carrier with amalgam.

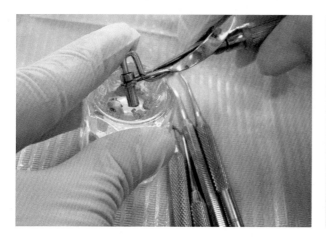

5. Dappen dish

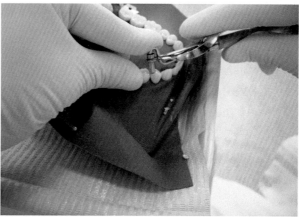

6. Unload the amalgam on the prepared cavity.

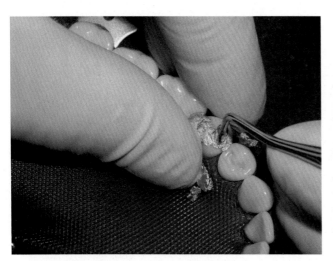

7. Condense the amalgam first with small condenser and then use larger condenser with firm pressure.

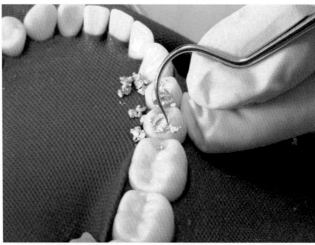

8. Remove the access amalgam with explorer.

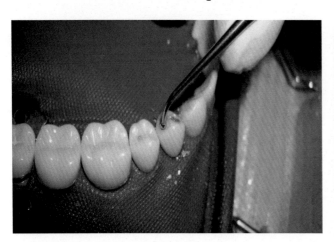

9. Burnish the occlusal surface with ball burnisher to bring the excess mercury to the surface and for more adaptation.

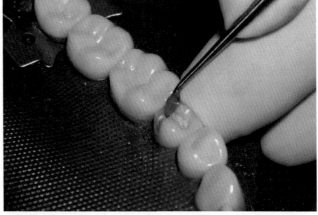

10. Carve the amalgam surface to create the occlusal anatomy using discoid-cleoid carver.

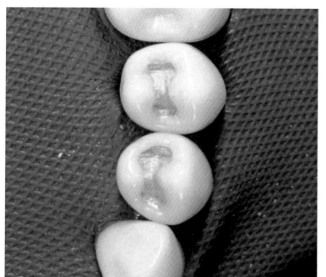
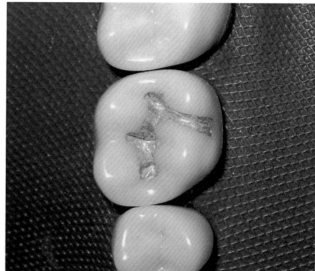

Final Stage after Carving and Burnishing

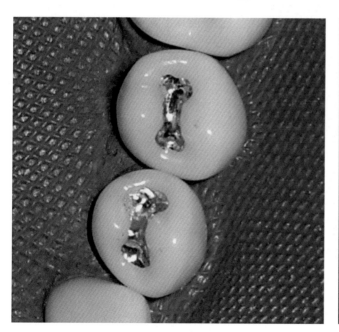
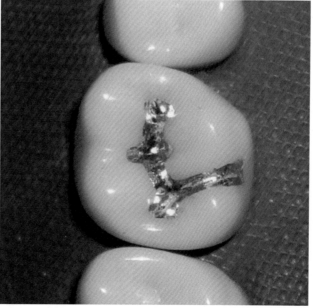

Polishing amalgam can be accomplished after twenty-four hours
or according to the manufacturer's instructions.

Classical Class I Cavity Preparation for Amalgam Restoration in Maxillary Premolars

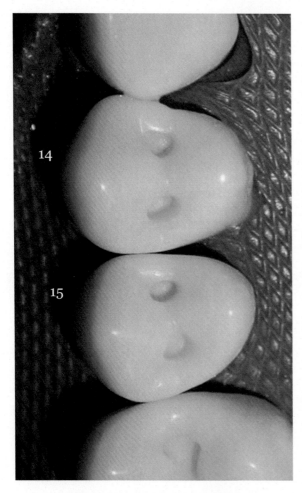

Occlusal Preparation Intact Transverse Ridge

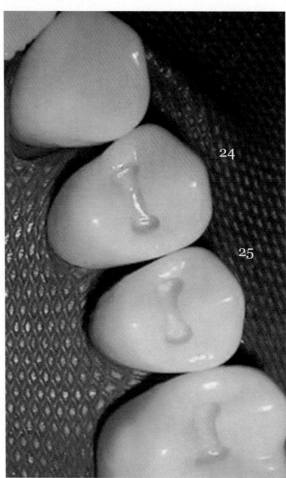

Occlusal Preparation Including the Transverse Ridge

Classical Amalgam Restoration for Class I Cavity Preparaton in Maxillary Premolars

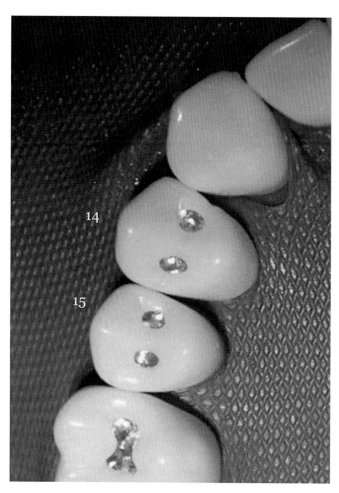

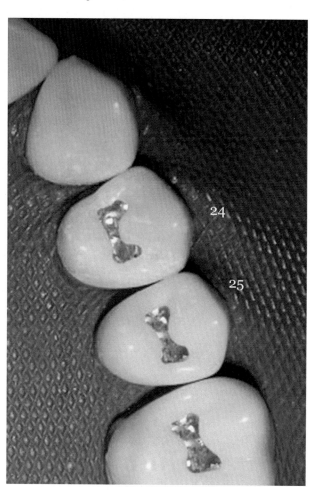

**Amalgam Restoration
Intact Transverse Ridge**

Occlusal Amalgam Restoration

Classical Class I Cavity Preparation for Amalgam Restoration in Maxillary Molars

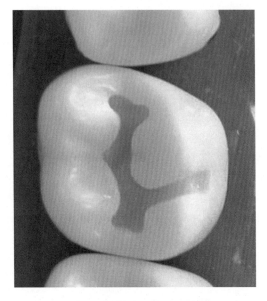

#16 Occlusal Cavity Preparation with Palatal Extension Including the Oblique Ridge

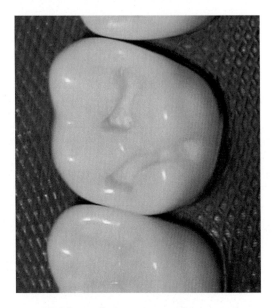

Occlusal Preparation #16 with Palatal Extension and Intact Oblique Ridge

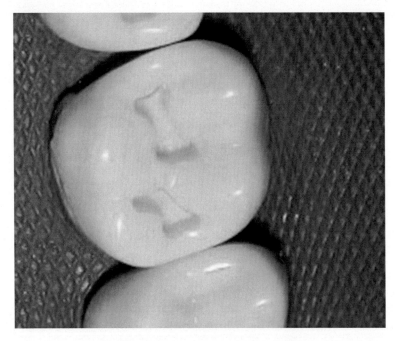

Occlusal Preparation #26 Intact Oblique Ridge without Palatal Extension

Classical Amalgam Restoration for Class I Cavity Preparation in Maxillary Molars

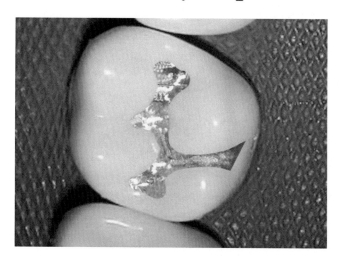

Occlusal Amalgam #16 with Palatal Extension

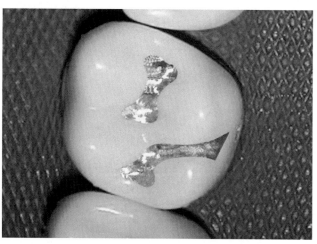

Occlusal Amalgam #16 with Palatal Extension Intact oblique ridge

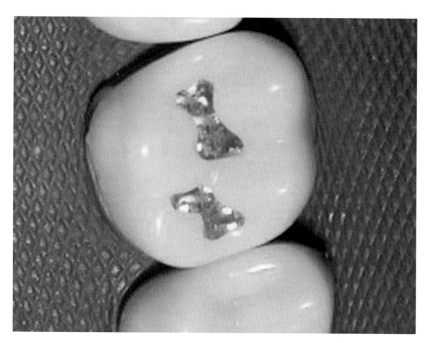

Occlusal Amalgam #26 Intact Oblique Ridge

Classical Class I Cavity Preparation for Amalgam Restoration in Mandibular Premolars

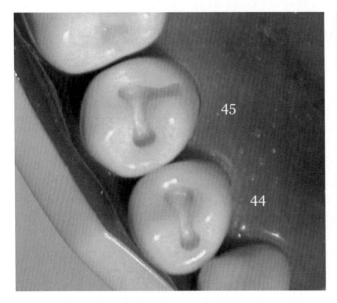

Occlusal Preparation in #45 with Lingual Extension

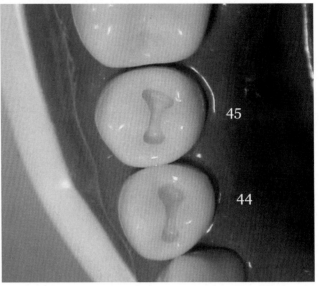

Occlusal Preparation Including the Transverse Ridge

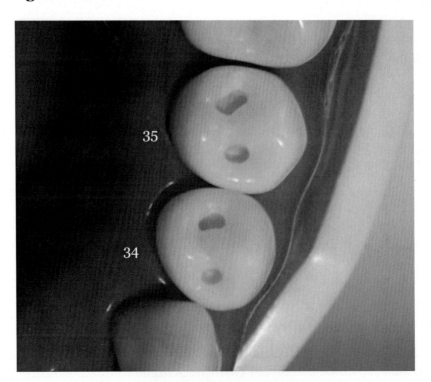

Occlusal Preparation The Transverse Ridge Is Intact.

Classical Amalgam Restoration for Class I Cavity Preparation in Mandibular Premolars

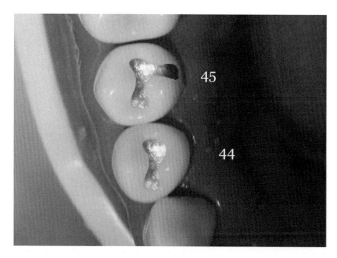

Occlusal Preparation in #45 with Lingual Extension

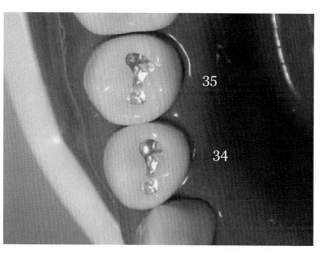

Occlusal Preparation Including the Transverse Ridge

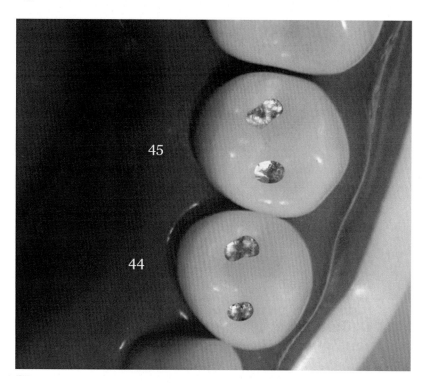

**Occlusal Preparation
The Transverse Ridge Is Intact.**

Classical Class I Cavity Preparation for Amalgam Restoration in Mandibular Molars

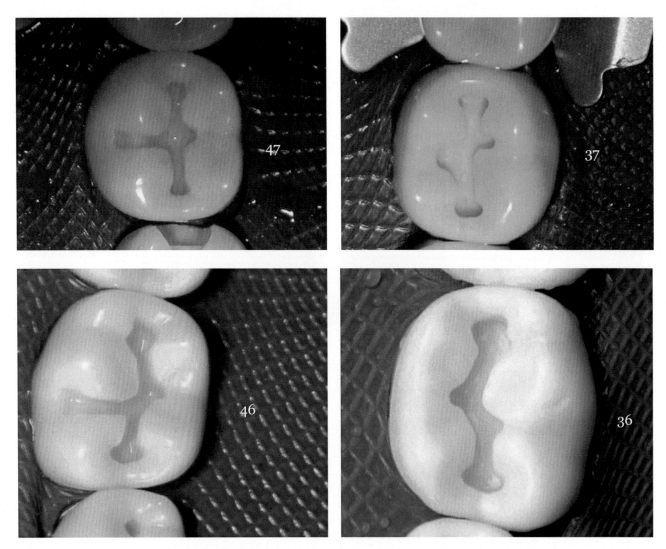

Occlusal Preparation with Buccal Extension

Occlusal Preparation

Classical Amalgam Restoration for Class I Cavity Preparation in Mandibular Molars

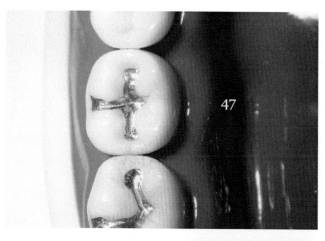 47

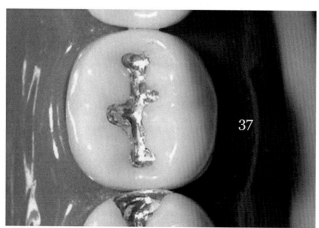 37

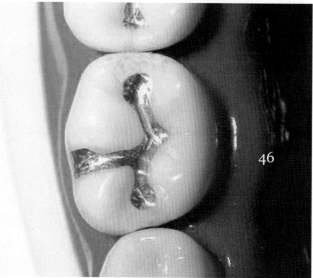 46

36

Occlusal Amalgam with Buccal Extension

Occlusal Amalgam

Classical Class I Buccal Pit Preparation and Restoration in Mandibular Molars

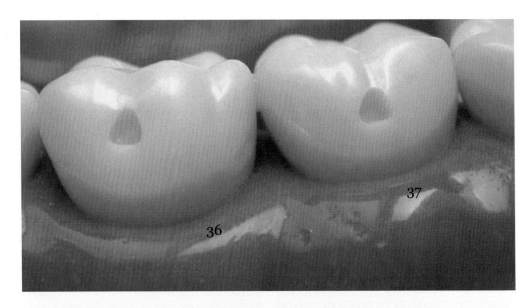

36   37

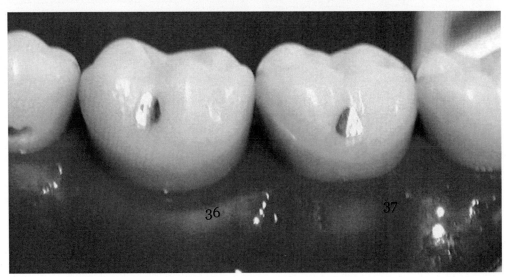

36   37

Cavity Preparation for Preventive Resin Restoration (PPR or Sealant)

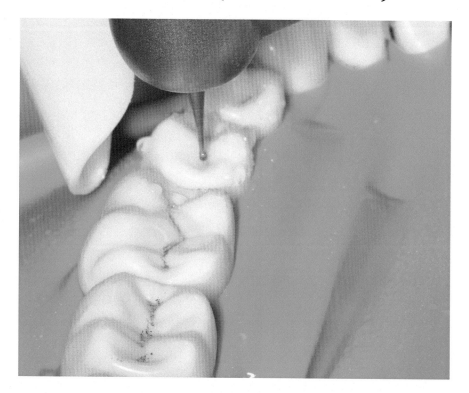

Remove Caries on Pit/Fissures Using Small Round Bur
Minimal Cavity Preparation Only

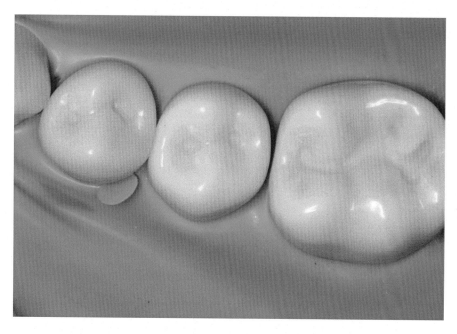

Final Preparation for PPR Restoration

Armamentarium for Preventive Resin Restoration (PRR or Sealant)

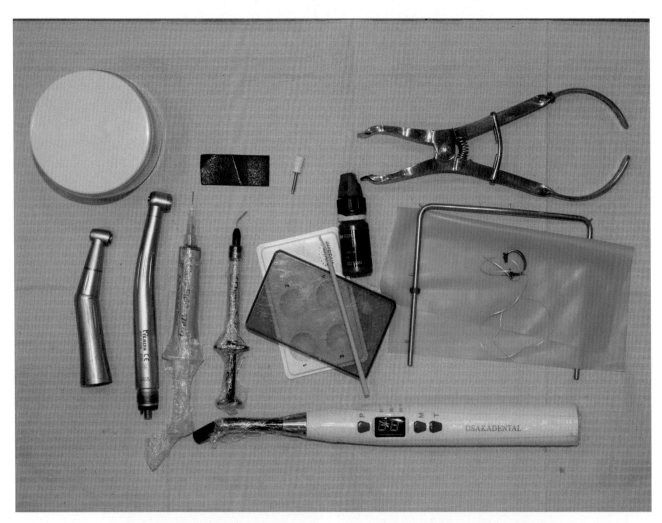

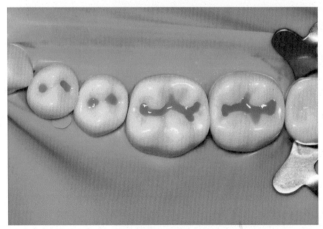

Etch the prepared cavity for fifteen to twenty seconds and then wash and dry.

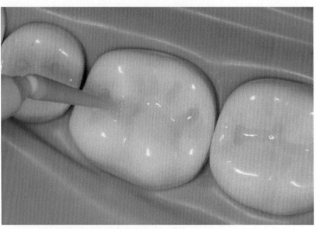

Using small brush, apply bonding agent on prepared cavity for twenty seconds and apply air for five seconds before curing.

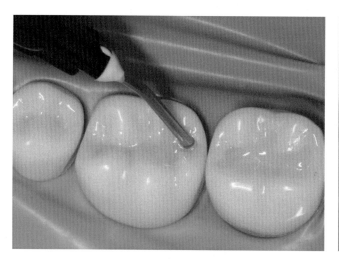

Fill the cavity with flowable composite.

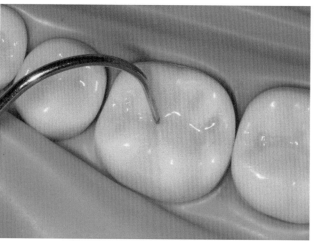

Use explorer to remove the bubbles and to fill the cavity evenly.

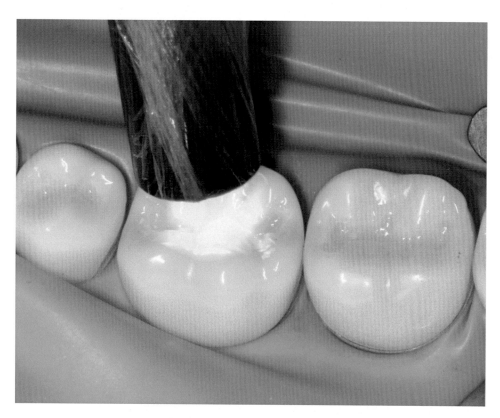

Light cure for twenty to forty seconds.

Cavity Preparation for Preventive Resin Restoration

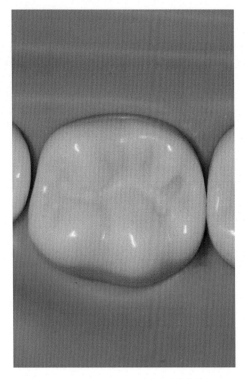

#36 PRR Cavity Preparation

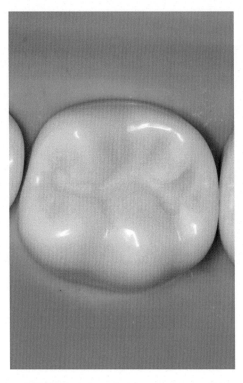

#37 PRR Cavity Preparation

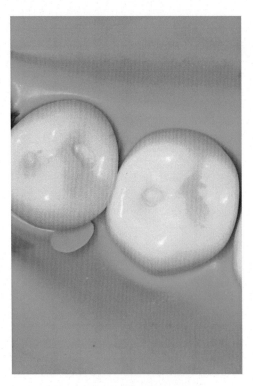

**#34 #35 PRR Cavity
Preparation with Intact
Transverse Ridge**

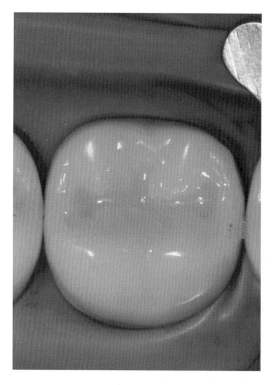

#36 PRR

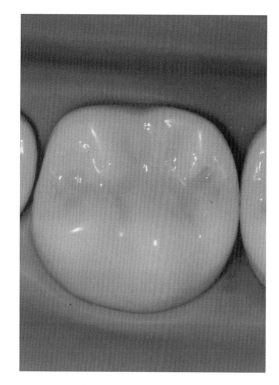

#37 PRR

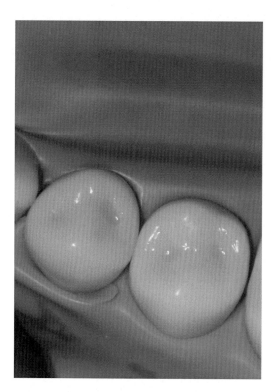

**#34, #35 PRR Composite
Intact Transverse Ridge**

Cavity Preparation for Class I Composite Restoration

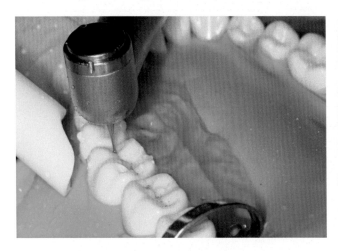

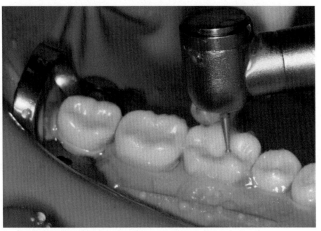

Make small dots on the deepest fissure/fossa first and then connect them to create the cavity outline.

Establish proper depth and width as for caries extension amalgam preparation, with no sharp angle and less extension for prevention

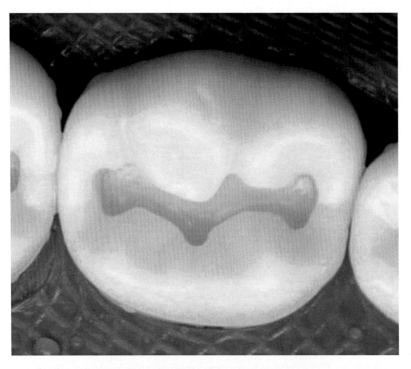

Class I Cavity Preparation

Armamentarium for Composite Restoration

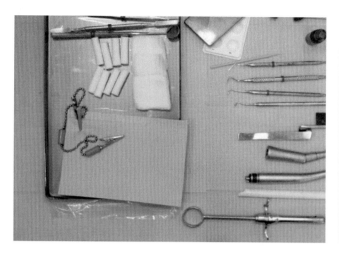
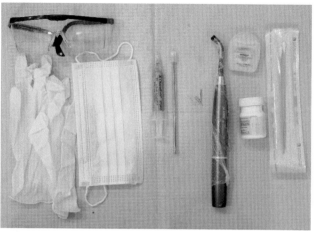

Composite Restoration Procedure for Class I Cavity Preparation

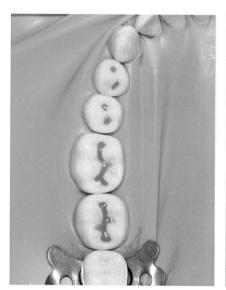
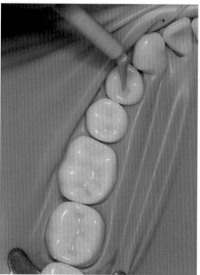

Etch the prepared cavity for fifteen to twenty seconds and then wash and dry.

Using a small brush, apply bonding agent on prepared cavity with gentle pressure and then distribute the excess bonding with dry air.

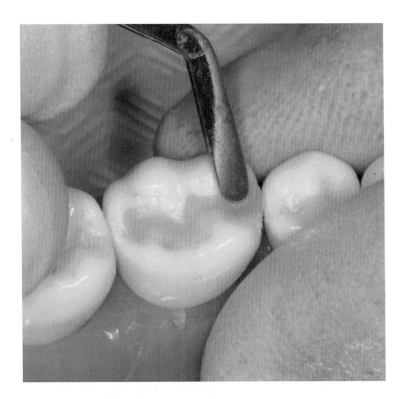

Apply the first increment of the composite.

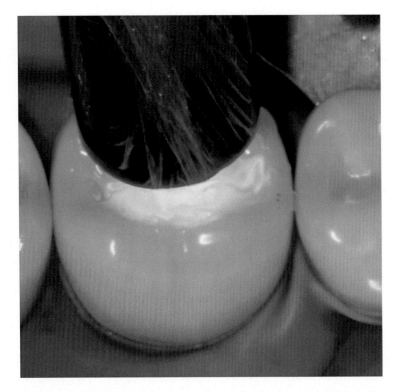

Light cure for minimum of twenty seconds each increment.

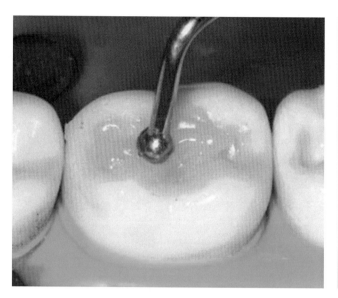

Fill the cavity with composite and use ball burnisher to condense and smoothen the surface and then cure.

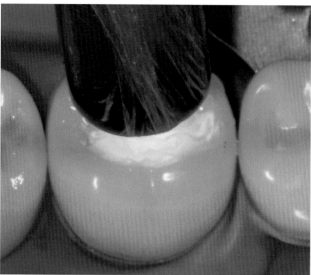

Light cure for twenty seconds.

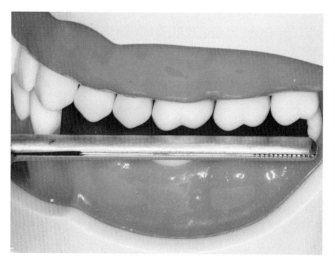

Check the occlusal for high points.

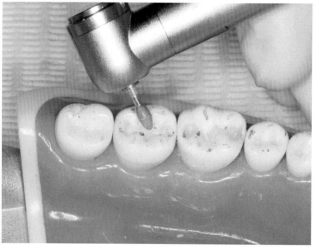

Adjust the occlusal surface using the finishing burs.

Classical Class I Cavity Preparation for Composite Restoration in Mandibular Premolars

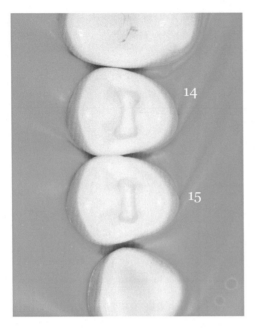

Occlusal Preparation, Including Transverse Ridge

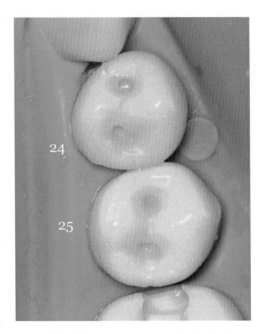

Occlusal Preparation Intact Transverse Ridge

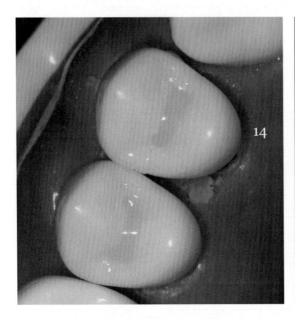

Occlusal Composite Restoration

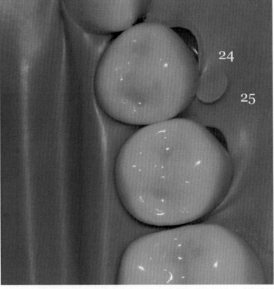

Composite Restoration Intact Transverse Ridge

Classical Class I Cavity Preparation for Composite Restoration in Maxillary Molars

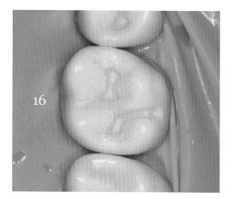
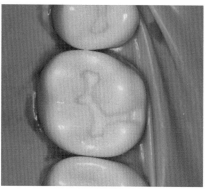
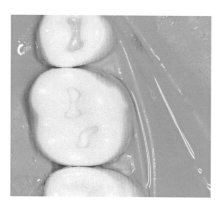

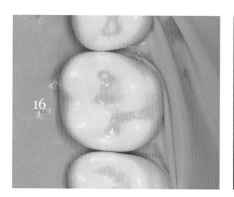
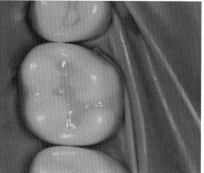
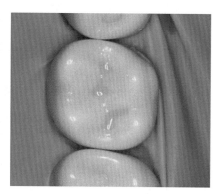

Classical Class I Cavity Preparation for Composite Restoration in Mandibular Molars

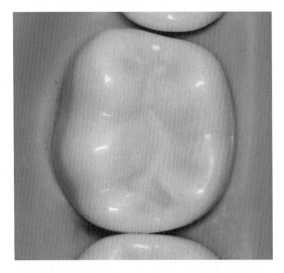

Simple Occlusal Preparation #36

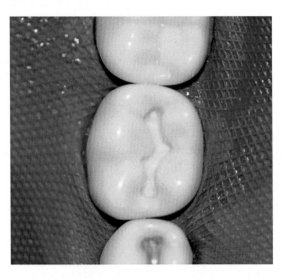

Classical Occlusal Preparation #46

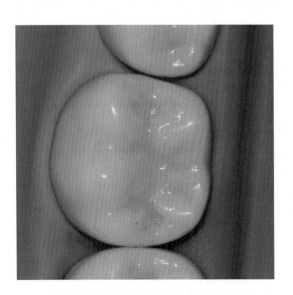

Occlusal Composite #36

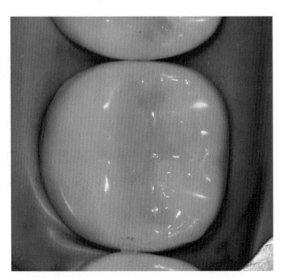

Occlusal Composite #46

Differences in Class I Cavity Preparation between Composite and Amalgam Restoration

CHARACTERISTICS	AMALGAM	COMPOSITE
Outline	Extension for prevention	Follow the caries only
Depth	1.5–2 mm	Follow the caries only
Width	One-quarter to one-third the intercuspal distance	Follow the caries only
Occlusal convergence	Important for retention	No need
Retentive features	Important in large cavity	Important in large cavity
Unsupported enamel	Remove	Don't remove in less stress area

Class II Cavity Preparation

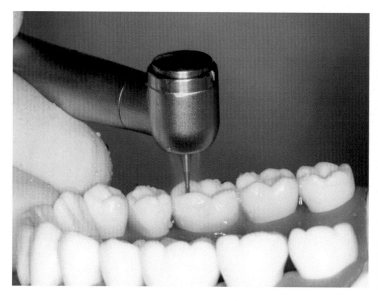 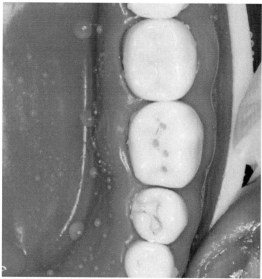

For beginners, mark small dots in the deepest fossa and fissures to create the outline of the cavity using appropriate small bur and then connect them with the same depth and width of the bur.

Bur Orientation

It is important during dental procedures treatment to orient the burs to be with the long axis of the tooth crown and perpendicular to the occlusal surface.

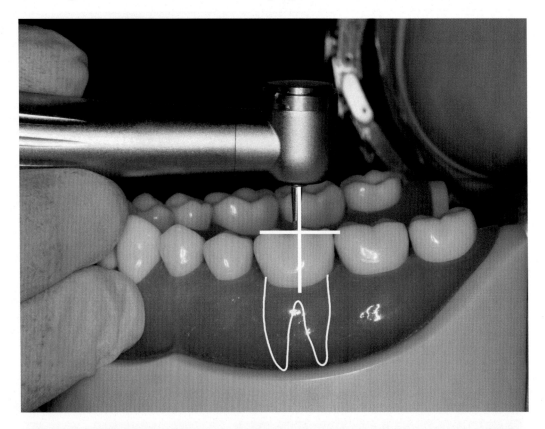

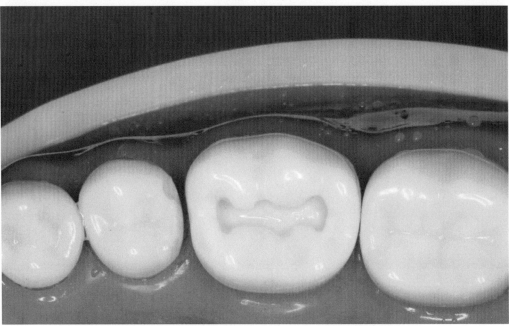

Finalised Class I Cavity Outline

Steps in Creating a Proximal Box in Class II

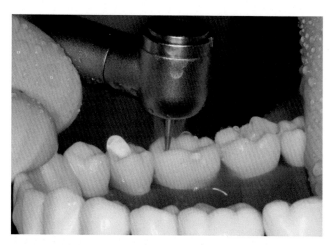

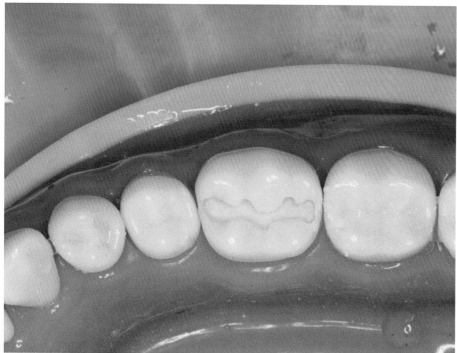

Extend the occlusal preparation towards the carious proximal marginal ridge having the same depth of the occlusal part.

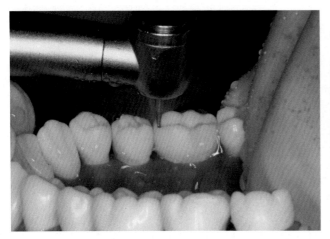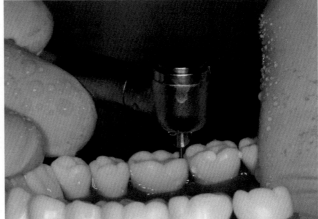

Prepare the proximal box by cutting deeper 0.5-1mm on the area of marginal ridge or as deep as the carious lesion extends without breaking the proximal contact.

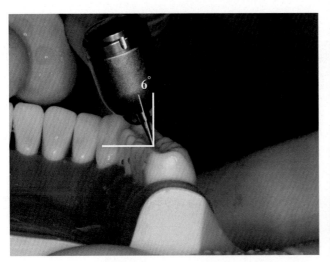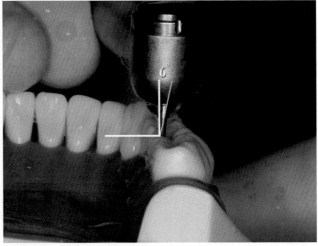

Create convergence occlusally and divergence proximally for resistance and retention features without breaking the contact.

Steps for Breaking a Proximal Contact Using Hand Instruments (e.g., Gingival Marginal Trimmer)

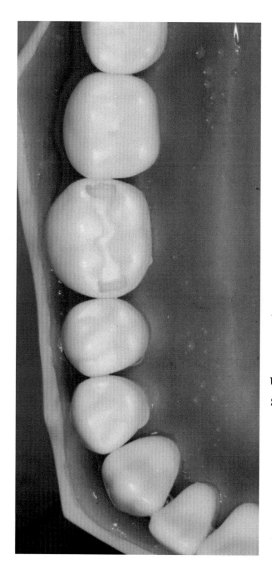

With gentle and firm pressure, use the gingival margin trimmer or any suitable hand instrument with side pressure to remove the remaining unsupported tooth structure to create the proximal box.

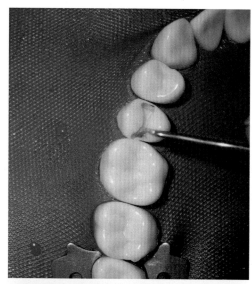

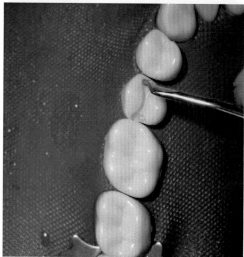

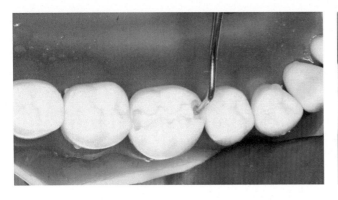 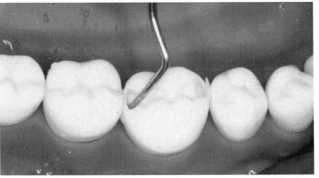

You can also use a spoon excavator instead of a gingival marginal trimmer.

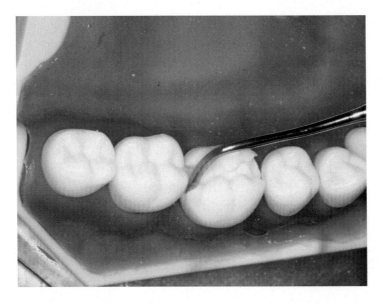

Smooth the gingival floors using a hatchet or gingival margin trimmer.

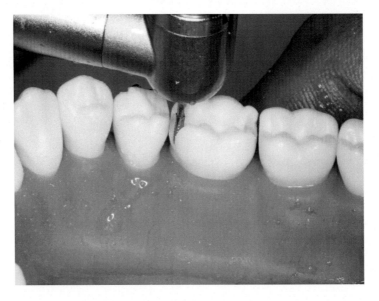

Flatten and smooth the gingival floor using a slow-speed Fissure bur.

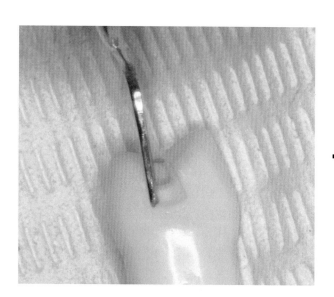

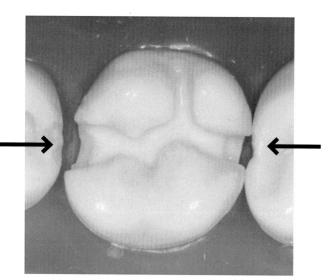

Removing Unsupported Enamel in the
Axial Walls Using a Hatchet Instrument

X Be careful not to injure the adjacent tooth.

Final Class II Cavity Preparation

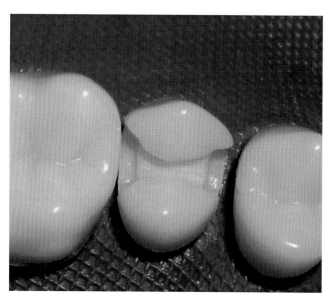

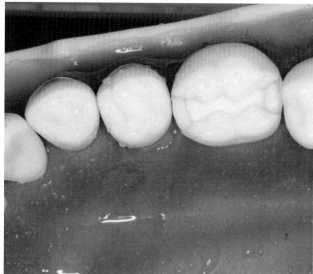

Preparing the Matrix Band in Class II

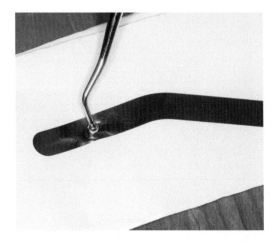

Burnish the band to compensate for the convexity of the proximal walls using the ball burnisher over a thick paper pad.

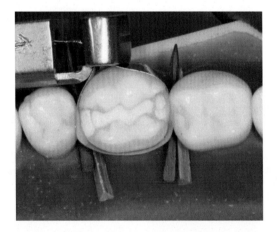

Place the matrix band and retainer supported with wooden wedge as explained in chapter 4.

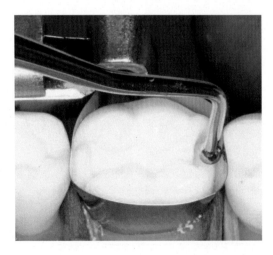

Contour the matrix band using the ball burnisher.

Steps for Amalgam Restoration in Class II Cavity Preparation

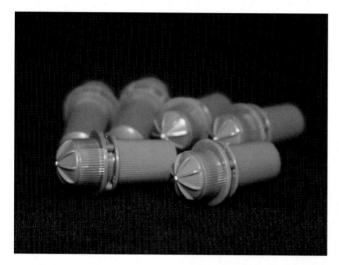

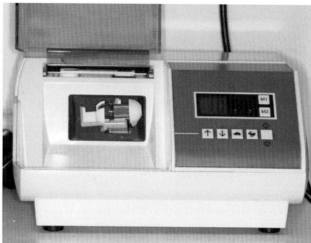

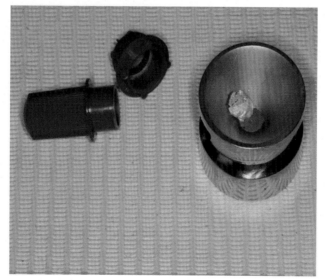

Activate the amalgam using amalgamator, as per manufacturer instructions.

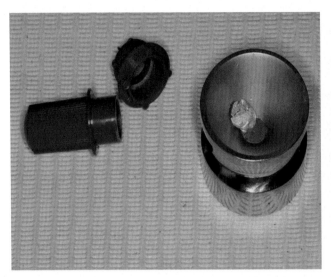

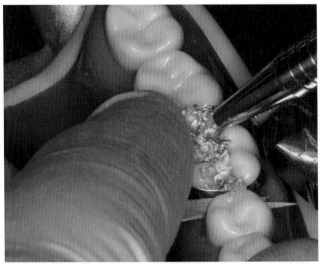

Release the activated amalgam on the well.

Load the amalgam carrier with amalgam to release it in the prepared cavity.

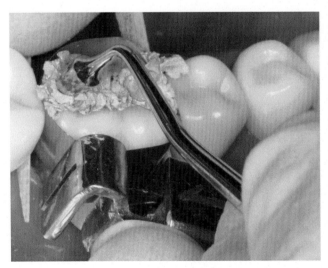

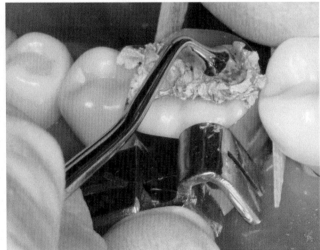

Condense the first amalgam increment with small condenser.

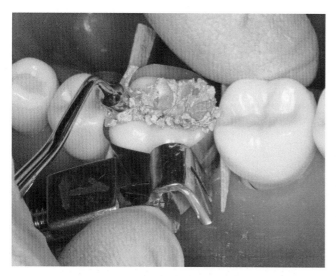

Condense more amalgam into cavity walls using larger condenser with firm pressure.

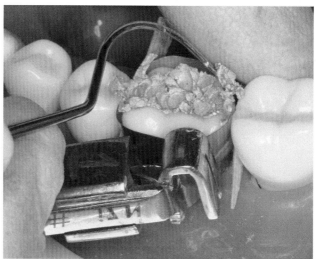

Remove the excess amalgam from the matrix band with explorer.

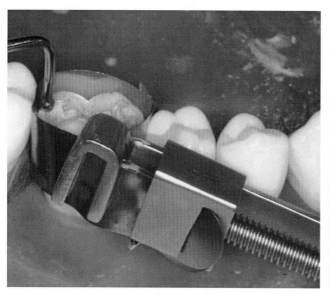

Burnish the occlusal surface with ball burnisher to adapt the amalgam and to bring the excess mercury to the surface.

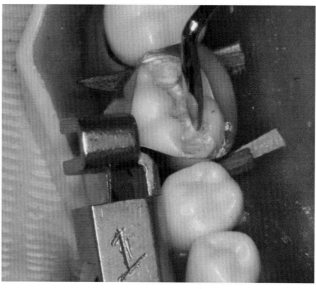

Contour and carve the interproximal anatomy using Hollenback carver.

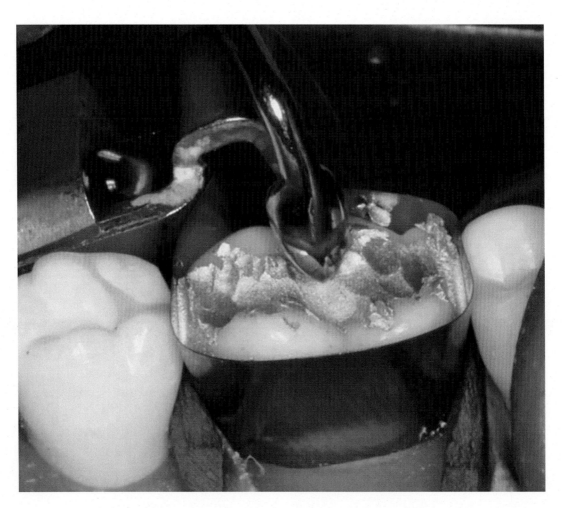

Create the occlusal anatomy using discoid cleoid carver.

How to Remove Matrix Band Retainer without Breaking the Proximal Amalgam Filling

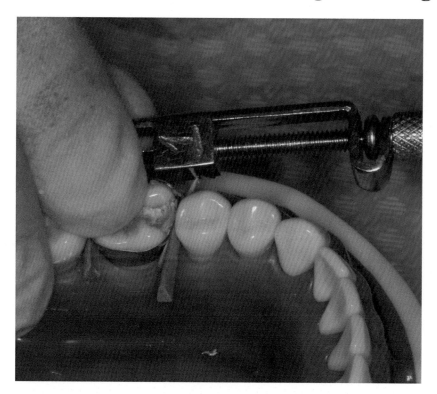

Support the retainer with one hand.

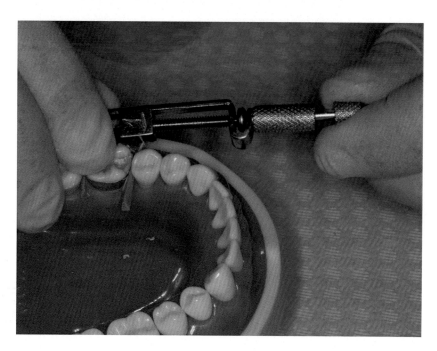

Unscrew the matrix retainer while supporting the head of the retainer.

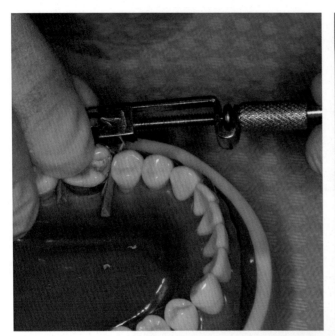
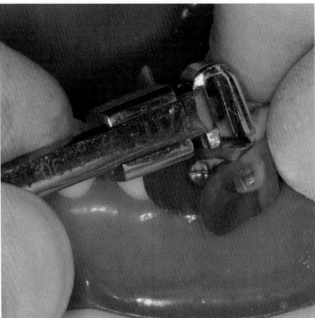
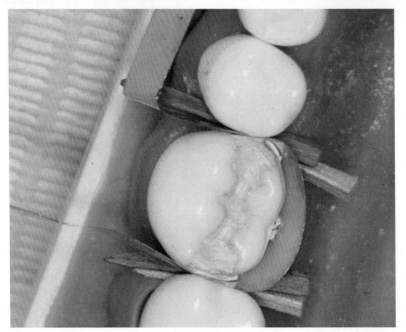

Support the band while releasing the retainer from the band.

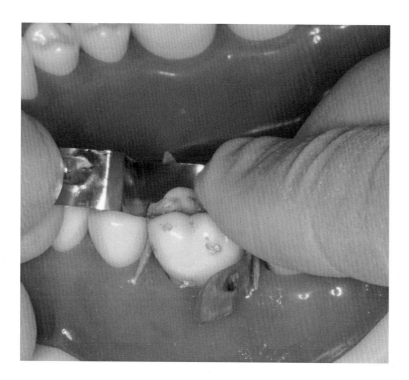

Gently remove one side of the band while placing your finger on the other side.

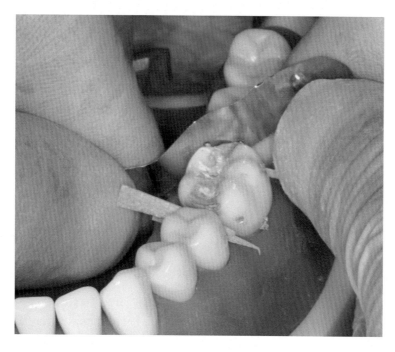

Hold both sides of the band and remove it in oblique direction lingually or buccally.

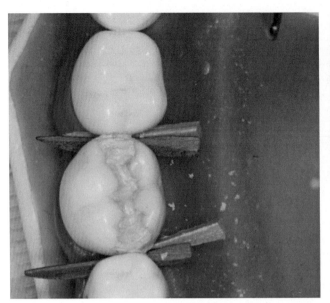 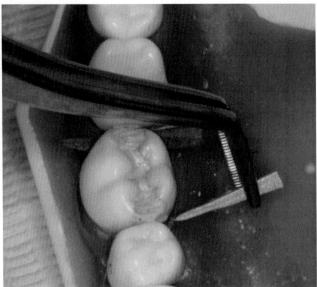

Remove the wooden wedge.

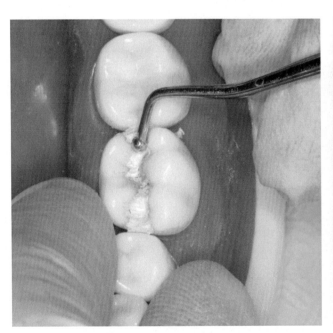

Burnish the amalgam surface.

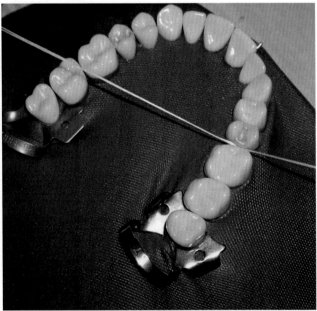

Check the proximal contact using dental floss. Little resistance while removing the floss is the sign of good proximal contact.

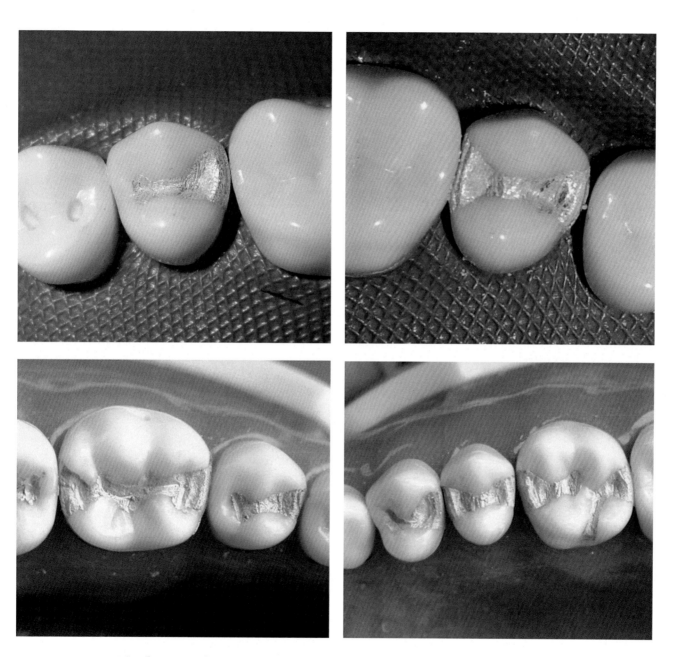

Final stage after carving different Class II amalgam restorations.

Classical Class II Cavity Preparation for Amalgam Restoration in Maxillary Premolars

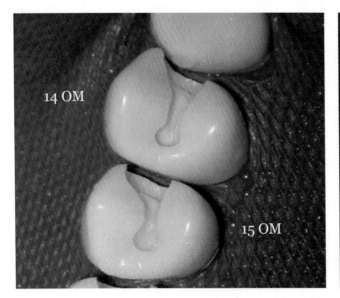

OM Preparation

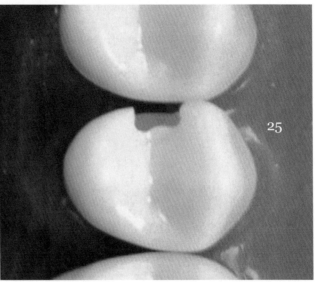

#25 M Box Preparation Only

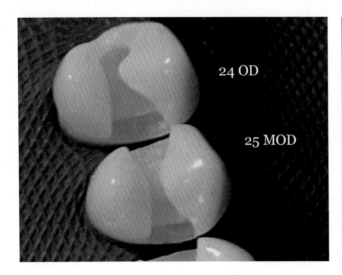

#15 OM Preparation Intact Transverse Ridges

Classical Amalgam Restoration for Class II
Cavity Preparation in Maxillary Premolars

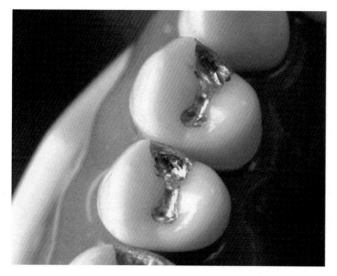

OM Amalgam Restoration

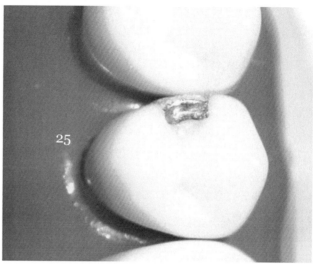

Amalgam Restoration Box Only

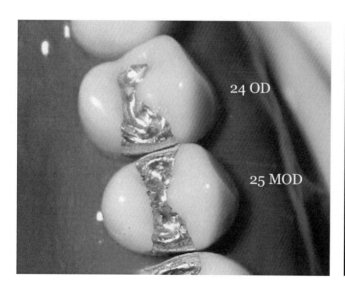

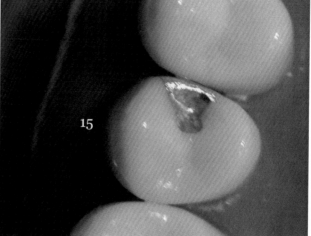

**OM Amalgam Intact
Transverse Ridge**

Classical Class II Cavity Preparation for Amalgam Restoration in Mandibular Premolars

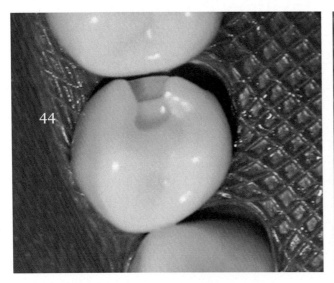

#44 OD Preparation Intact Transverse Ridge

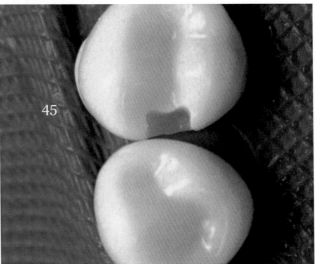

#45 M Box Preparation Only

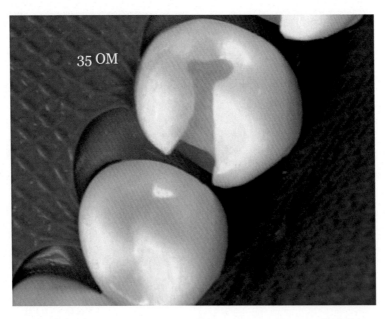

OM Preparation Including Transverse Ridge

Classical Amalgam Restoration for Class II Cavity Preparation in Mandibular Premolars

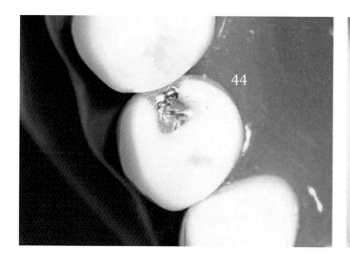
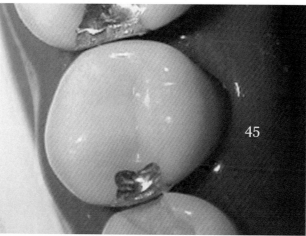
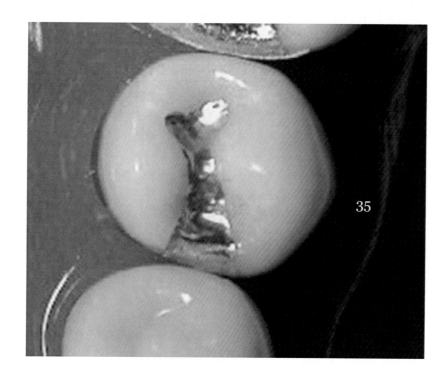

Classical Class II Cavity Preparation for Amalgam Restoration in Maxillary First Molars

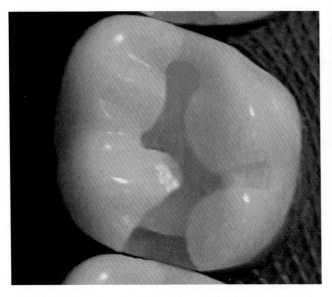

#16 OD Class II with Palatal Extension

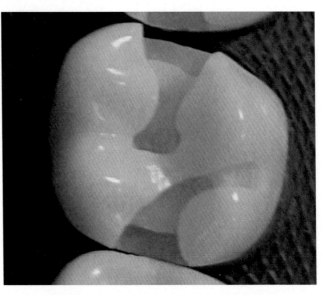

#16 MOD Class II Intact Oblique Ridge with Palatal Extension

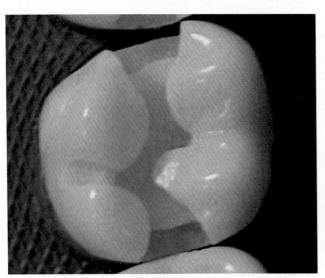

#26 MOD Class II with Palatal Extension

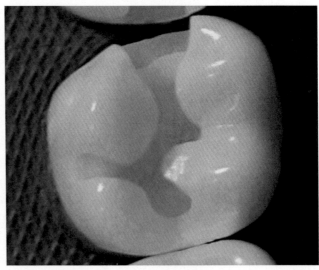

#26 OM Class II with Palatal Extension

Classical Class II Amalgam Restoration in Maxillary First Molars

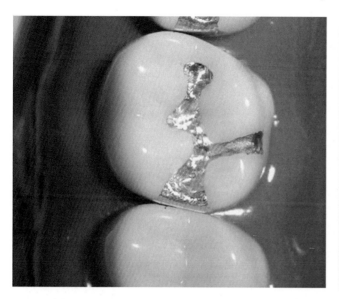

#16 OD Class II with Palatal Extension

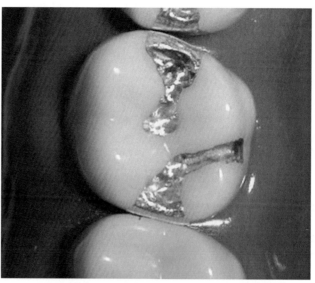

#16 MOD Class II Intact Oblique Ridge with Palatal Extension

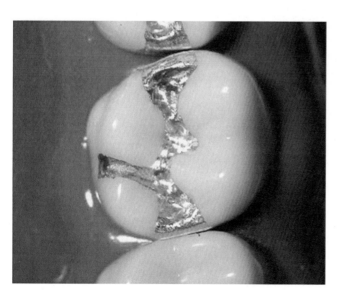

#26 MOD Class II with Palatal Extension

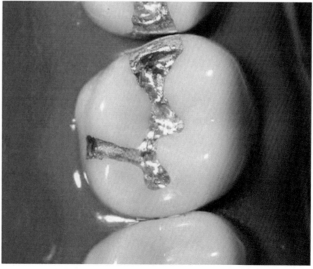

#26 OM Class II with Palatal Extension

Classical Class II Cavity Preparation for Amalgam Restoration in Mandibular First Molars

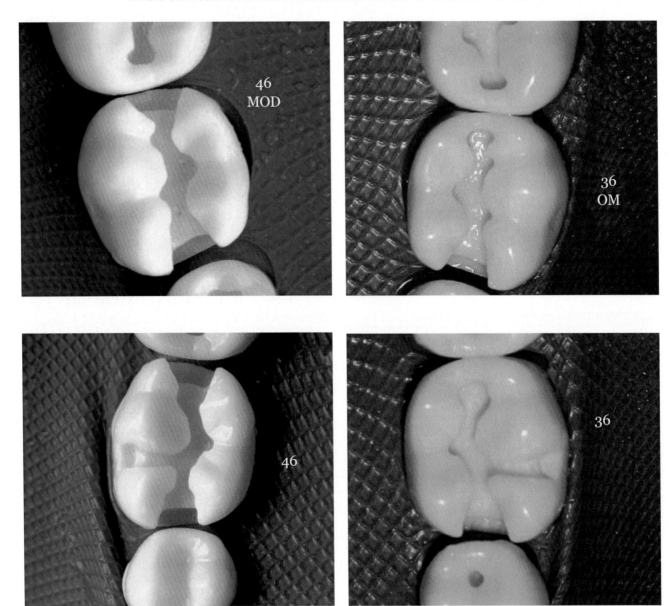

46
MOD

36
OM

46

36

Classical Amalgam Restoration for Class II Cavity Preparation in Mandibular First Molars

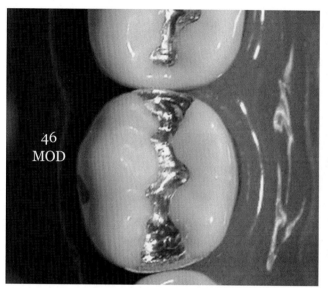
46
MOD

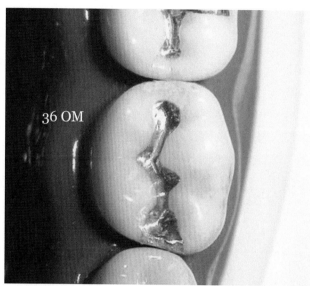
36 OM

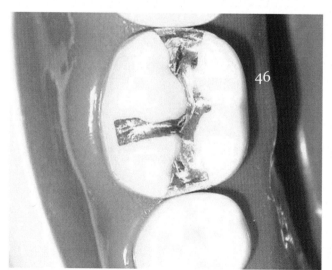
46

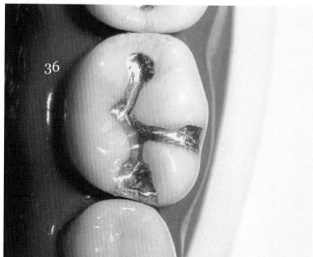
36

Classical Class II Cavity Preparation for Composite Restoration in Mandibular Molars

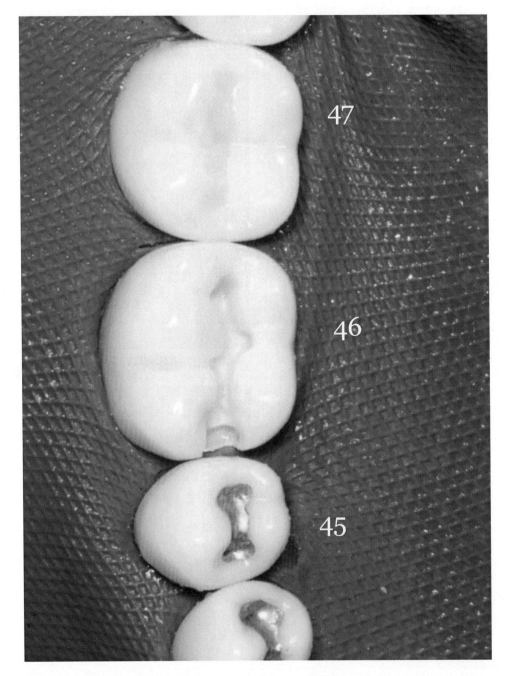

#46 OM Preparation

Classical Composite Restoration for Class II Cavity Preparation in Mandibular Molars

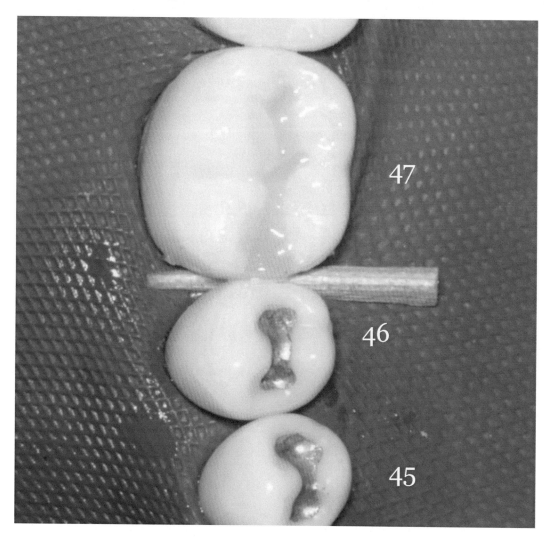

#46 OM Composite Restoration

Classical Class II Cavity Preparation for Composite Restoration in Mandibular First Molars

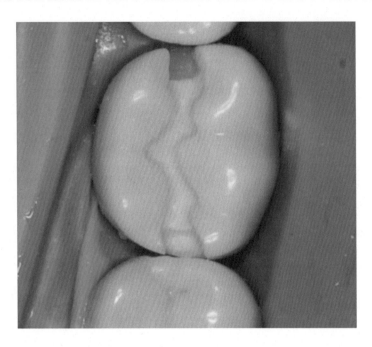

#36 MOD Preparation

Classical Composite Restoration for Class II Cavity Preparation in Mandibular First Molars

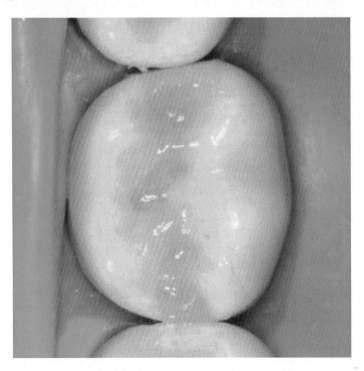

#36 MOD Composite Restoration

Classical Class II Cavity Preparation for Composite Restoration in Mandibular Premolars

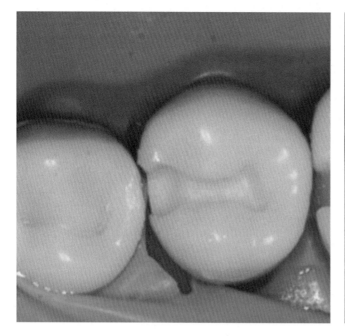

#45 OM Cavity Preparation Including Transverse Ridge

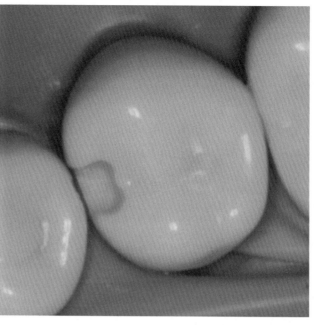

#45 M Box Cavity Preparation Only

Classical Composite Restoration for Class II in Mandibular Premolars

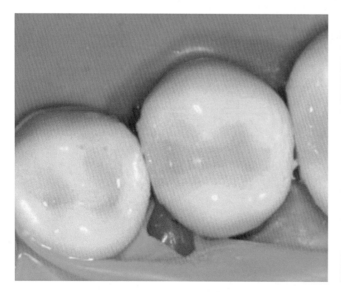

#45 OM Composite Restoration including transverse ridge

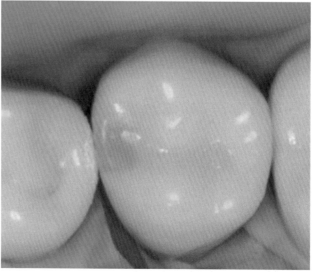

#45 M Box Composite Restoration only

Classical Class II Cavity Preparation for Composite Restoration in Maxillary Molars

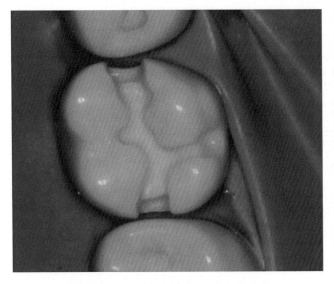

#26 MOD Cavity Preparation with Lingual Extension

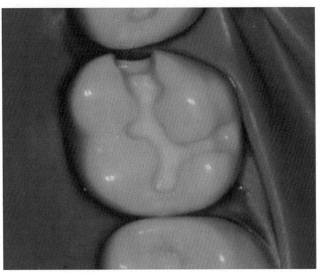

#16 OM Cavity Preparation

Classical Composite Restoration for Class II Cavity Preparation in Maxillary Molars

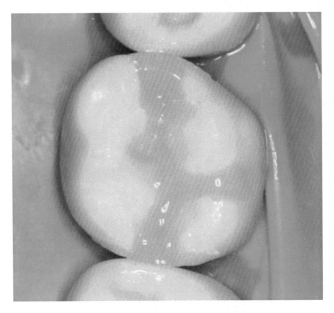

#26 MOD Composite Restoration with Lingual Extension

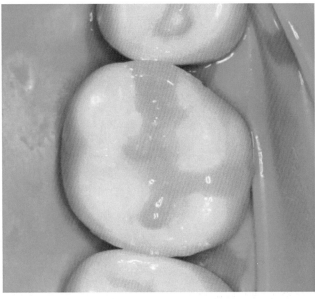

#16 OM Composite Restoration

Classical Class II Cavity Preparation for Composite Restoration in Maxillary Premolars

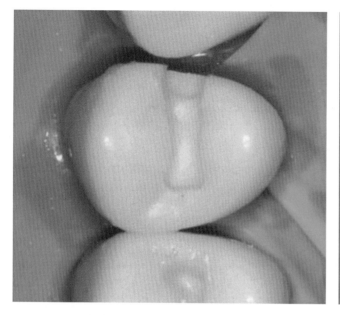

#15 OM Cavity Preparation

#25 Box only preparation

Classical Composite Restoration for Class II Cavity Preparation in Maxillary Premolars

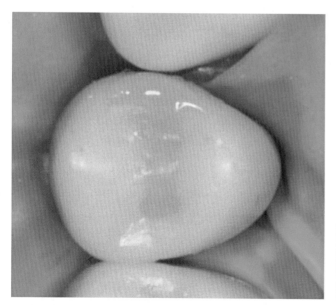
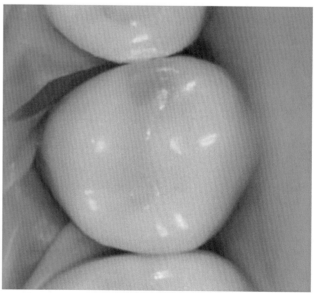

#15 OM Composite Restoration

#25 Box only composite restoration

Differences between Amalgam and Composite Cavity Preparation

CHARACTERISTICS	AMALGAM	COMPOSITE
Outline	Extension for prevention	Follow the caries only
Depth	1.5–2 mm	Follow the caries lesion
Width	One-quarter to one-third the intercuspal distance	Follow the caries only
Occlusal convergence	Important for retention	Needed in large cavity
Retentive features	Important in large cavity	Important in large cavity
Unsupported enamel	Remove	Don't remove in less stress area
Proximal clearance	Important	Not important

Classical Class III Cavity Preparation
for Composite Restoration

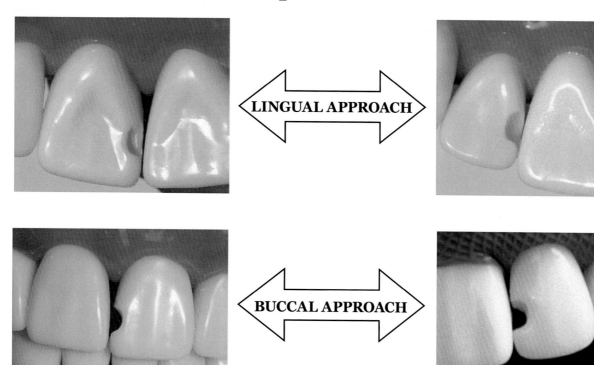

LINGUAL APPROACH

BUCCAL APPROACH

Classical Composite Restoration for
Class III Cavity Preparation

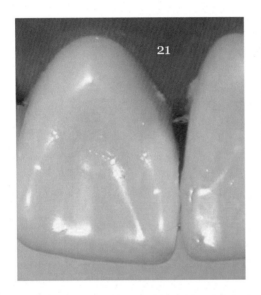

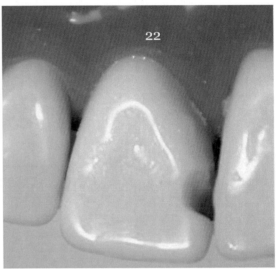

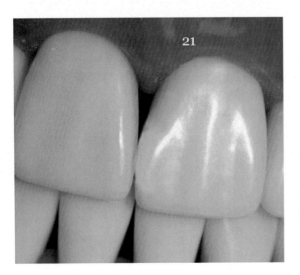

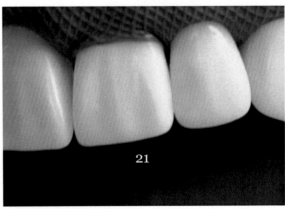

Cavity Preparation for Class III Composite Restoration

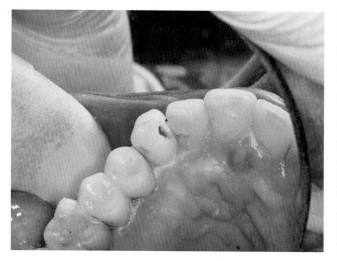

Lingual approach preparation. Bur should be perpendicular to enamel surface, and initial opening made close to adjacent tooth. With the same bur used, enlarge the opening for removal of caries.

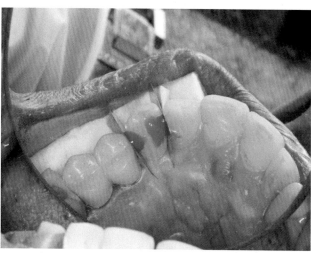

Clear sectional matrix or piece of metal matrix band should be placed between cavity and the adjacent tooth. Acid etch for fifteen to twenty seconds or as recommended by the manufacturer.

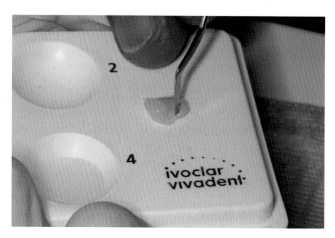

Choose the shade of composite to be used. Apply the bonding agent and cure for maximum of forty seconds. Apply the first increment into the cavity, and use the small ball burnisher to condense the composite inside the prepared cavity.

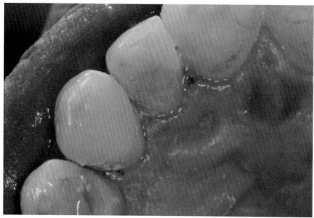

Dry the cavity and then apply the composite using the carrier on the prepared cavity, starting with box first.

Class III Cavity Preparation and Composite Restoration Buccal Approach

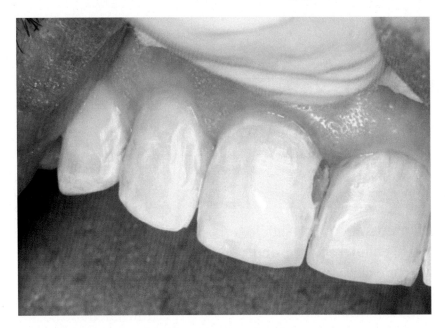

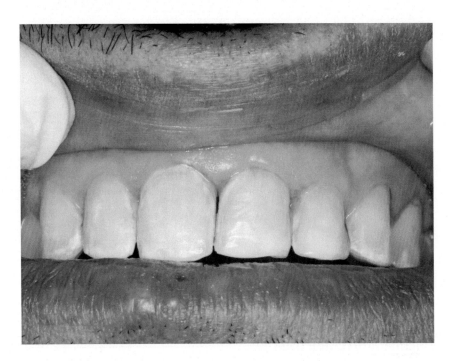

Class IV Cavity Preparation

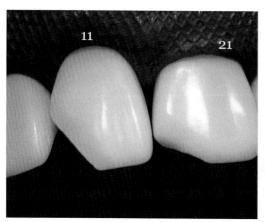 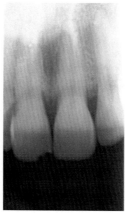 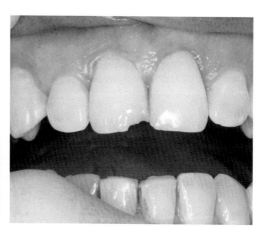

Class IV Composite Restoration

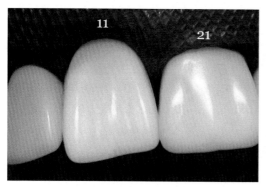 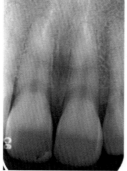 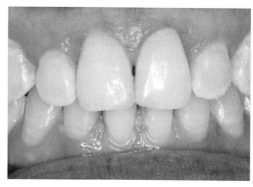

CLASS V CAVITY PREPARATION FOR AMALGAM RESTORATION IN MANDIBULAR PREMOLARS

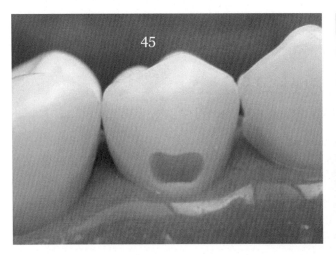
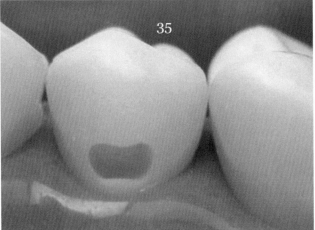

Class V Amalgam Restoration in Mandibular Premolars

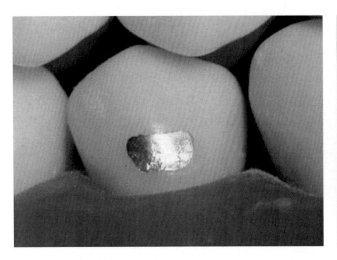
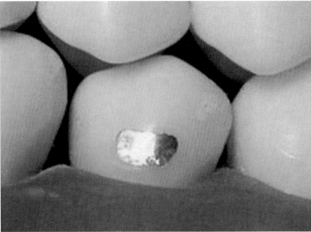

CLASS V CAVITY PREPARATION FOR COMPOSITE RESTORATION

Class V Composite Restoration

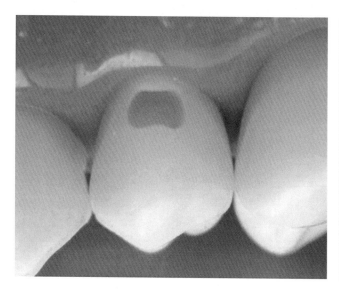

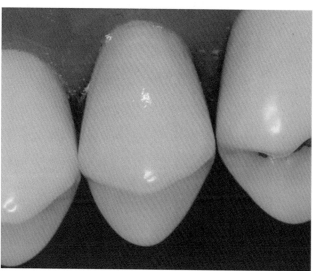

Class V Cavity Preparations and Their Corresponding Restorations

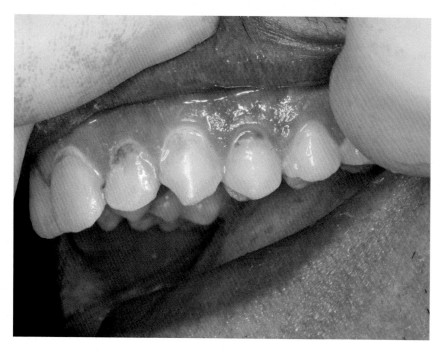

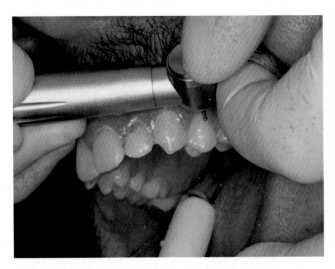

Remove the defect area of the
tooth using a small bur.

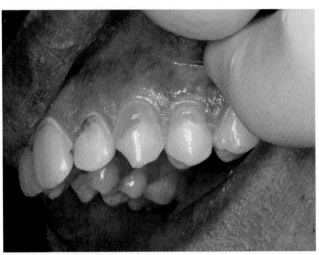

Etch for ten to fifteen seconds
and then wash and dry.

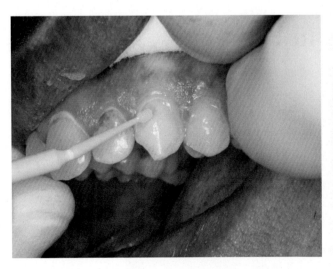

Apply bonding agent with smallest
brush and apply air for five seconds.

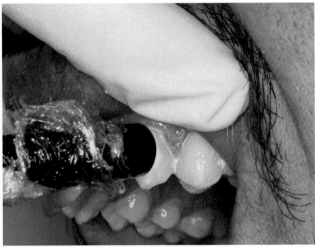

Cure for twenty to forty seconds.

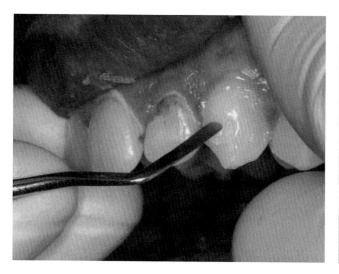

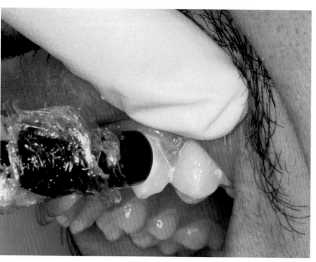

Select the appropriate shade and adapt the composite to the cavity with carful pressure.

Contour the composite before the light cure.

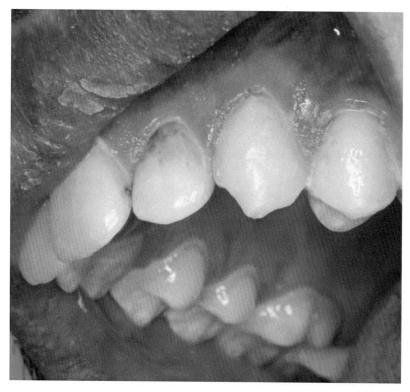

Composite Restoration Tooth #23, #24

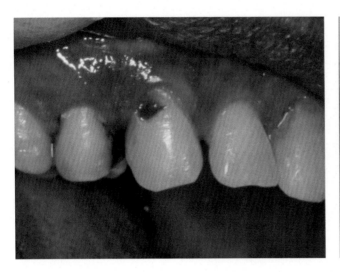
Cervical class V caries tooth #13

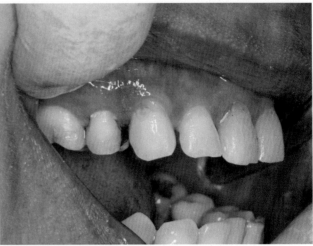
Class V cavity preparation tooth #13

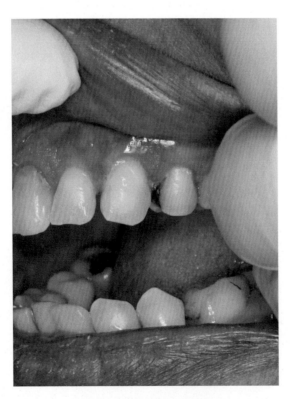
**Class V composite
restoration tooth #13**

Class VI Cavity Preparation for Amalgam Restoration

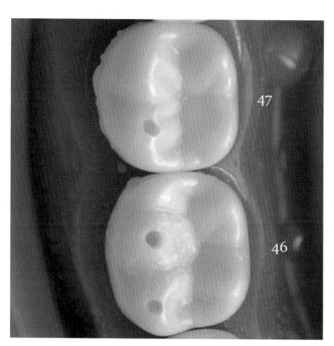

Class VI Amalgam Restoration

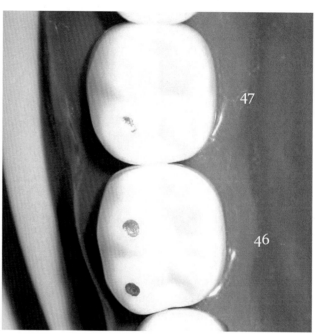

Class VI Cavity Preparation for Composite Restoration

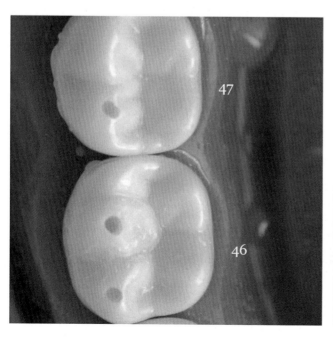

Class VI Composite Restoration

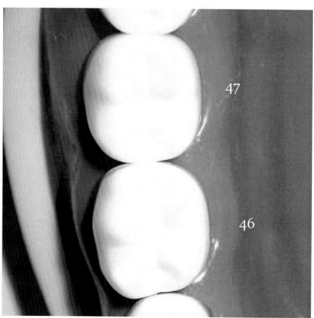

REFERENCES

1. Banerjee, Avijit, Watson, Timothy F. (2015), *Pickard's Guide to Minimally Invasive Operative Dentistry*, 10th edition, Oxford Medical Publication.
2. Heymann, Harald O., Swift, Edward J., and Ritter, Andre V. (2013), *Sturdevant's Art & Science of Operative Dentistry,* 6th edition, Elsevier.
3. Garg, Nisha, Garg, Amit (2013), *Textbook of Operative Dentistry*, 2nd edition, Jaypee Brothers Medical Publishers.
4. Hilton, Thomas J., Ferracane, Jack L., Broome, James C. (2013), *Summitt's Fundamentals of Operative Dentistry: A Contemporary Approach*, 4th edition, Quintessence Publishing Co.

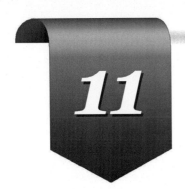

11

LABORATORY PROJECTS AND ASSESSMENT EXAMS

Best Practice and Training in Phantom Lab

Dental caries diagnosis has had many modifications and improvements. In this book, the classic G. V. Black caries lesion classification is our standard. Any other classification can be added by the lab's supervisor.

Teaching and phantom lab staff may discuss the cases systematically before the students start the restorative preparations and restorations.

Tasks have been designed to first ask a question, which allows discussion for diagnosis, and then the answer is on the next page.

Students must be familiar with such discussions, preparing them for the next clinical courses, treating the real patient's teeth. Remember, all cases have been selected to fulfill the phantom lab training courses.

This book is based on the standard cavity preparation recommended by most international operative dentistry references.

Some simulation steps can improve the training in the phantom lab, including taking the chief complaint of the patient (most chief complaint expected have been raised) and getting a history of chief complaints (can be discussed with students).

These diagnostic tools are used during clinical examinations:

- visual examination (discolouration or cavitation)
- radiographical examination (intraoral x-ray images-bite-wings and periapical).
- dental explorer (most of our cases propose catch or cavitation in the caries lesions)
- transillumination to discover the non cavitated caries lesion in anterior teeth.

Concluding the correct caries lesion diagnosis.

Restoring the caries lesion with suitable and available restorative material (amalgam and composite are the most common restoration used in the phantom lab or in the clinics).

Task No. 1

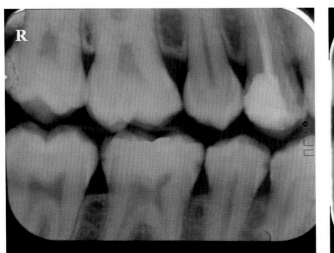
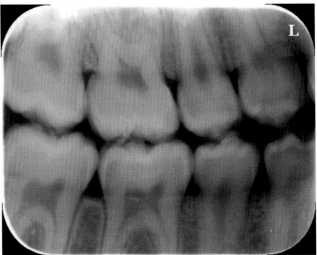

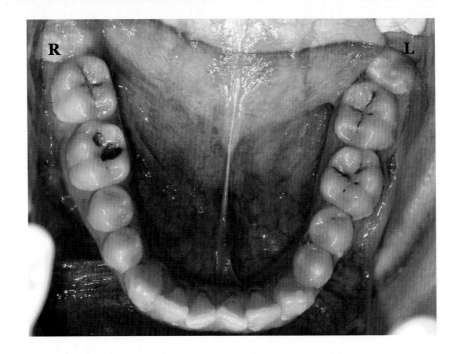

Patient Complaint
Slight pain with sweet food and cold drinks related to tooth #36.

What is the clinical diagnosis for tooth #36?
What is the expected treatment for this case?

Clinical Findings
Cavitated and discoloured occlusal pit and fissures.

Radiographical Findings
bite-wing radiograph shows slight or non-radiolucency under occlusal enamel.

Diagnosis: Tooth #36 is occlusal caries.
Treatment: Class I amalgam restoration or Class I composite restoration.

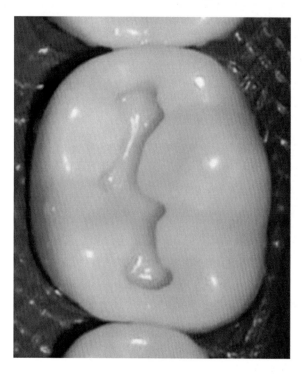

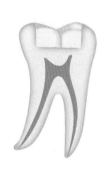

Ideal depth
1.5–2 mm

Ideal width
1-1.5mm or as
caries extends

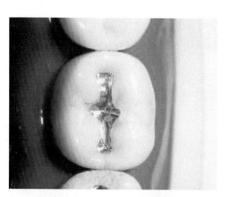

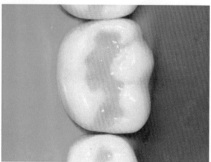

Task No. 2

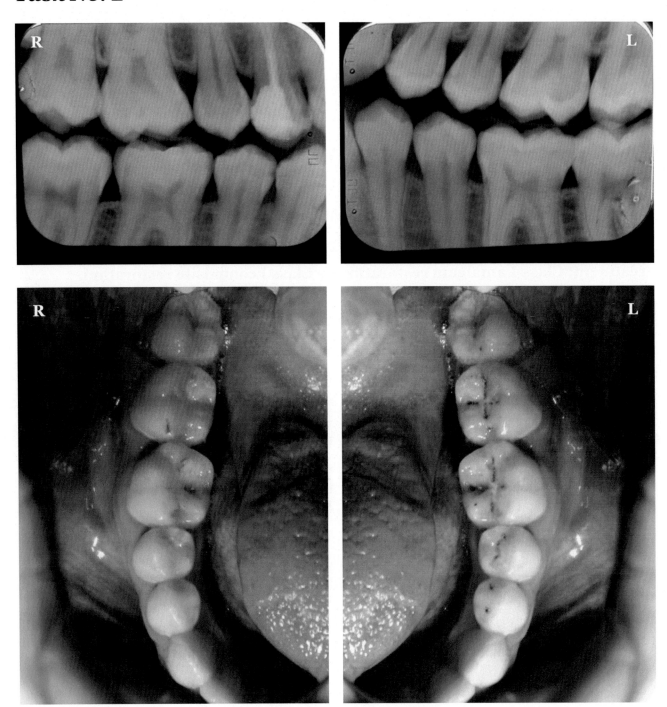

Patient Complaint
Slight pain with sweet food and cold drinks related to tooth #35.

What is the clinical diagnosis for tooth #35?
What is the expected treatment for this case?

Clinical Findings
Some black discolouration in the occlusal pit and fissures and white spot lesions more opaque when dried and disappear when wet with water.

Radiographical Findings
Bite-wing radiograph shows slight or non-radiolucency under occlusal enamel.

Diagnosis: Tooth #35 is occlusal caries.
Treatment: Class I amalgam restoration or Class I composite restoration

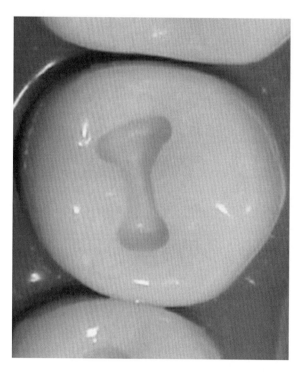

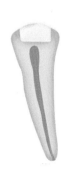

Ideal depth
1.5–2 mm

Ideal width
1-1.5mm or as
caries extends

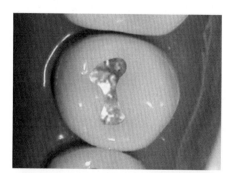

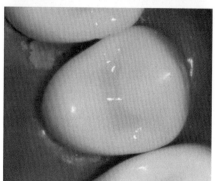

Task No. 3

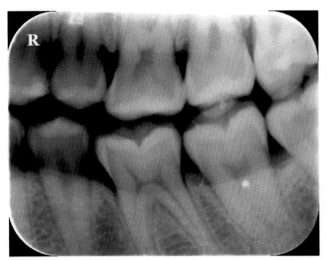
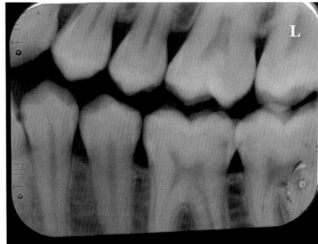

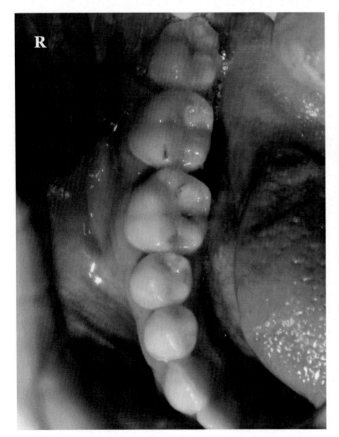
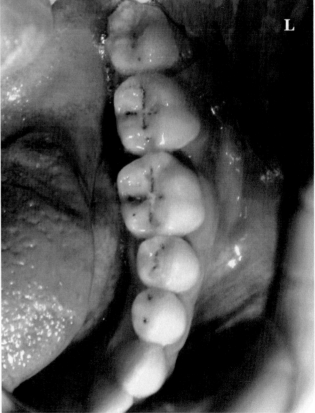

Patient Complaint
Slight pain with sweet food and cold drinks related to tooth #46.

What is the clinical diagnosis for tooth #46?
What is the expected treatment for this case?

Clinical Findings

Some black discolouration in the occlusal pit and fissures and white spot lesions more opaque when dried and disappear when wet with water.

Radiographical Findings

Bite-wing radiograph shows slight or non-radiolucency under occlusal enamel.

Diagnosis: Tooth #46 is occlusal caries.
Treatment: Class I amalgam restoration or Class I composite restoration.

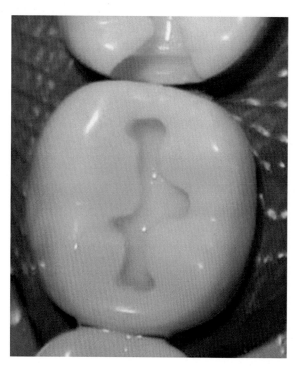

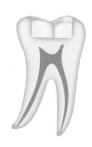

Ideal depth
1.5–2 mm

Ideal width
1-1.5mm or as
caries extends

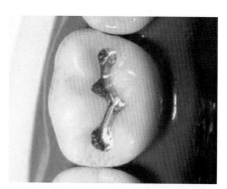

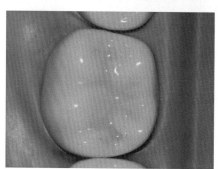

Task No. 4

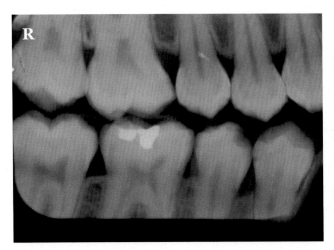
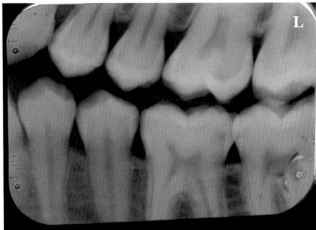

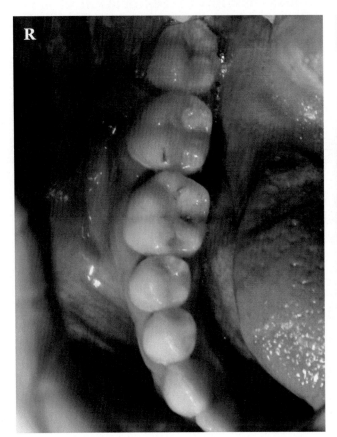
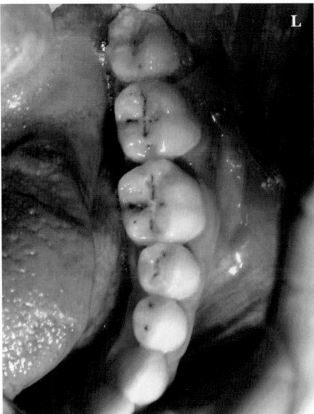

Patient Complaint
I had no pain but I want to check my teeth.

What is the clinical diagnosis for tooth #34?
What is the expected treatment for this case?

Clinical Findings

Small black discolouration in the occlusal pit with white spot lesions more opaque when dried and disappear when wet with water.

Radiographical Findings

Bite-wing radiograph shows slight or non-radiolucency under occlusal enamel.

Diagnosis: for tooth #34 is occlusal pit caries.
Treatment: Class I amalgam restoration or Class I composite restoration.

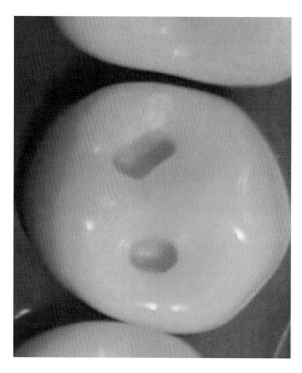

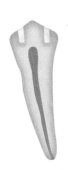

Ideal depth
1.5–2 mm

Ideal width
1-1.5mm or as
caries extends

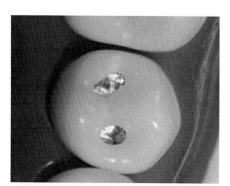

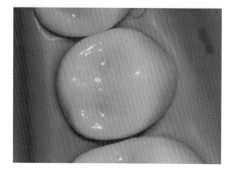

Task No. 5

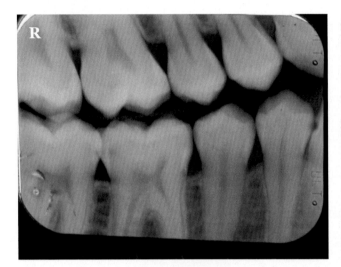
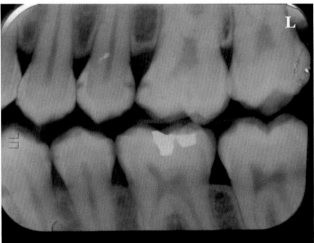

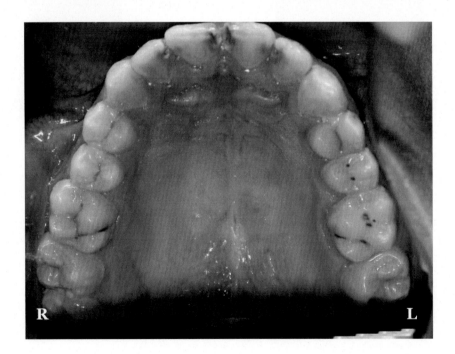

Patient Complaint
I had no pain but I want to check my teeth.

What is the clinical diagnosis for tooth #15?
What is the expected treatment for this case for tooth #15?

Clinical Findings

Small black discolouration in the occlusal pit with white spot lesions more opaque when dried and disappear when wet with water.

Radiographical findings :

Bite-wing radiograph shows slight or non-radiolucency under occlusal enamel.

Diagnosis: for tooth #15 is occlusal caries.
Treatment: Class I amalgam restoration or Class I composite restoration

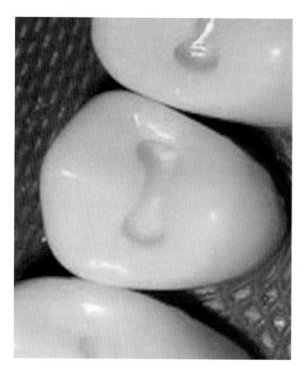

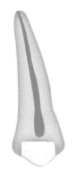

Ideal depth
1.5–2 mm

Ideal width
1-1.5mm or as
caries extends

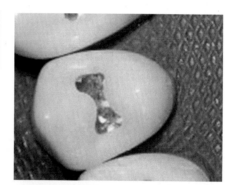

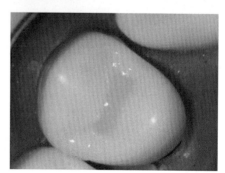

Task No. 6

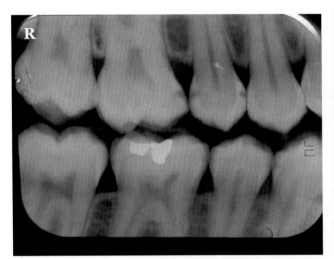
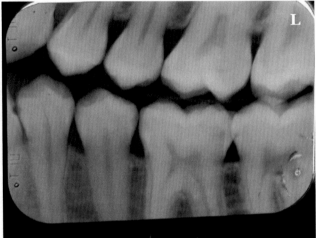

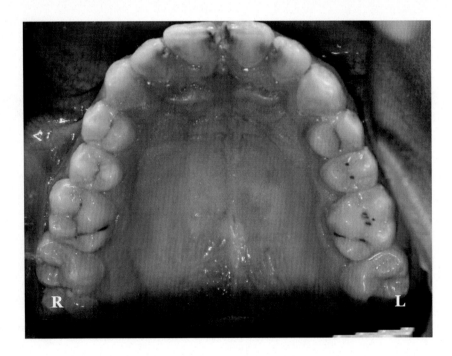

Patient Complaint

I had no pain but I want to check my teeth .

What is the clinical diagnosis for tooth #25?

What is the expected treatment for this case for tooth #25?

Clinical Findings
Small cavitated and black discolouration in the occlusal pit and intact transverse ridge tooth #25.

Radiographical Findings
Bite-wing radiograph shows no proximal caries.

Diagnosis: for tooth #25 is occlusal caries.
Treatment: Two separated pit amalgam restoration or composite restoration without jeopardise the transverse ridge.

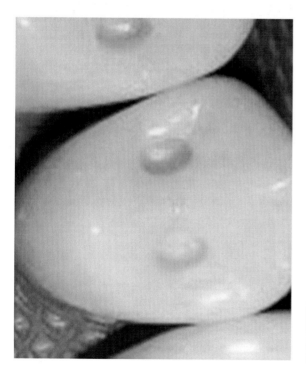

Ideal depth
1.5–2 mm

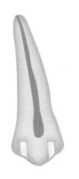

Ideal width
1-1.5mm or as
caries extends

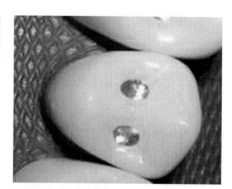

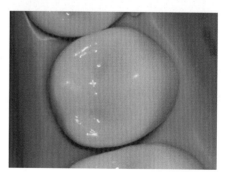

Task No. 7

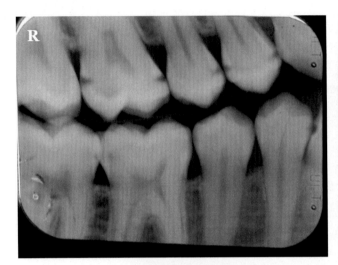
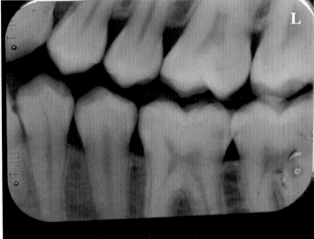

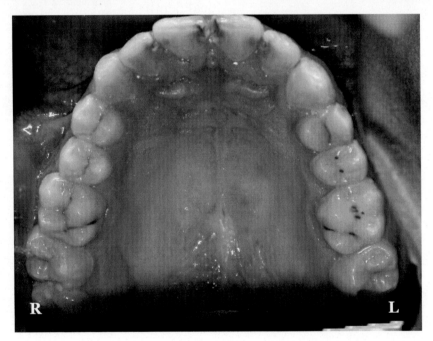

Patient Complaint
slight to moderate pain with sweet food and cold drinks related to tooth #26.

What is the clinical diagnosis for tooth #26?
What is the expected treatment for this case?

Clinical Findings

Cavitated black discolouration in the occlusal surface extending to the palatal pit and intact oblique ridge.

Radiographical findings :

Bite-wing radiograph shows no proximal caries but radiolucency under occlusal enamel.

Diagnosis: for tooth #26 is occlusal caries extending to the palatal pit in the distopalatal groove.
Treatment: Two separated occlusal amalgam or composite restoration without jeopardise the oblique ridge.

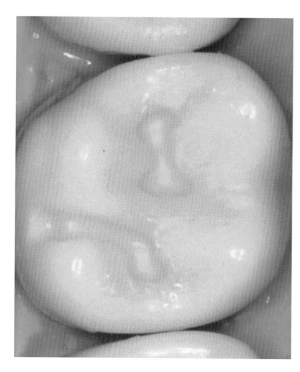

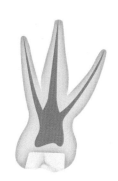

Ideal depth
1.5–2 mm

Ideal width
1-1.5mm or as
caries extends

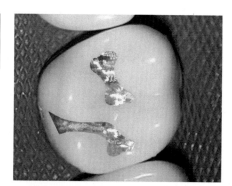

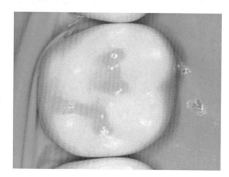

Task No. 8

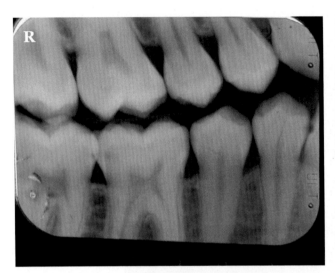

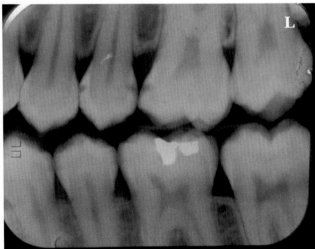

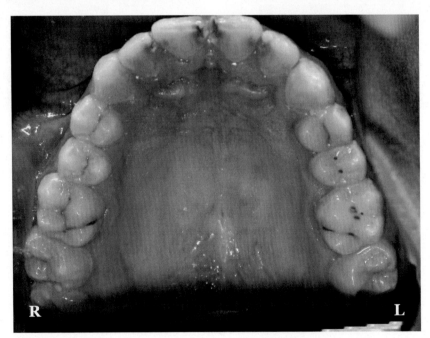

Patient Complaint
Slight to moderate pain with sweet food and cold drinks related to tooth #16.

What is the clinical diagnosis for tooth #16?
What is the expected treatment for this case?

Clinical Findings

Cavitated black discolouration in the occlusal surface extending to the palatal pit including the oblique ridge.

Radiographical Findings

Bite-wing radiograph shows no proximal caries but radiolucency under occlusal enamel.

Diagnosis: for tooth #16 is occlusal caries extending to the palatal pit in the distopalatal groove, including the oblique ridge.

Treatment: Occlusal (class I) amalgam or composite restoration including the oblique ridge.

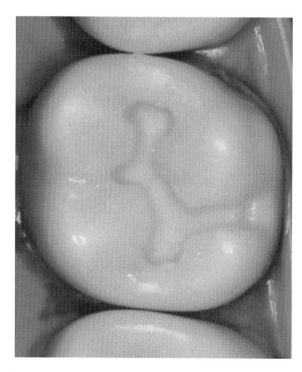

Ideal depth 1.5–2 mm

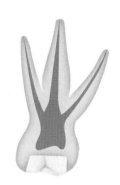

Ideal width 1-1.5mm or as caries extends

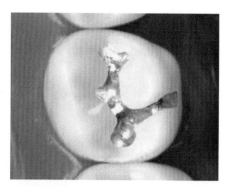

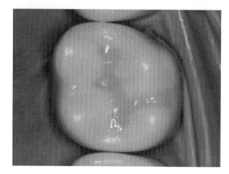

Task No. 9

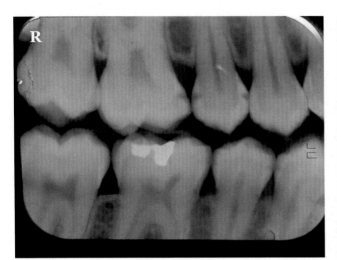
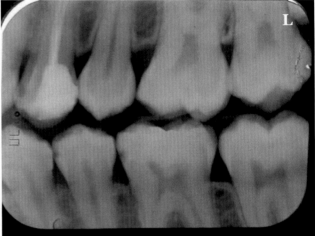

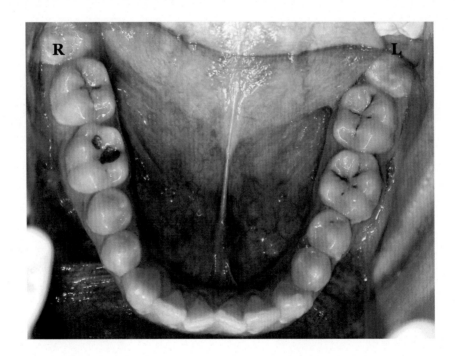

Patient Complaint
Reversible moderate pain with sweet food and cold drinks related to tooth #36.

What is the clinical diagnosis for tooth #36?
What is the expected dental restorations for this case?

Clinical Findings
Cavitated occlusal surface with black discolouration.

Radiographical Findings
Bite-wing radiograph shows small mesial radiolucency.

Diagnosis: for tooth #36 is occlusomesial OM caries lesion.
Treatment: Occlusomesial (class II OM) amalgam or composite restoration.

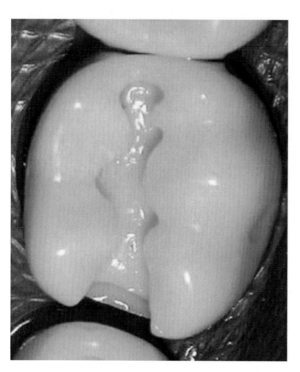

Ideal depth
1.5–2 mm

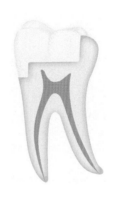

Ideal width
1-1.5mm or as
caries extends

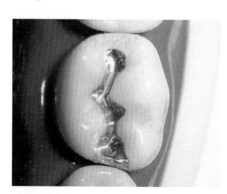

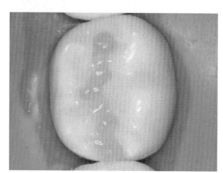

Task No. 10

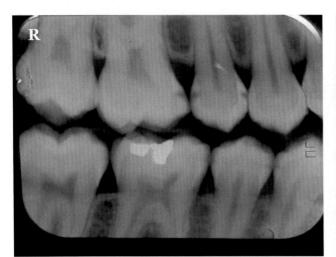
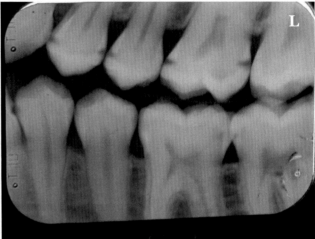
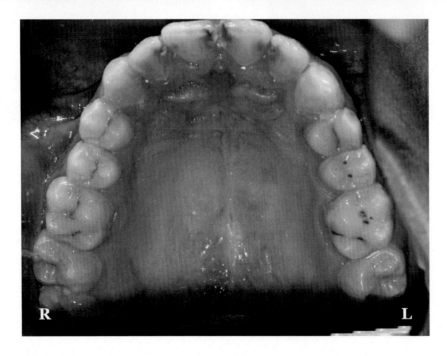

Patient Complaint
Reversible moderate to severe pain with sweet food and cold drinks related to tooth #26.

What is the clinical diagnosis for tooth #26?
What is the expected dental treatments for this case?

Clinical Findings

Cavitated black discolouration in the occlusal surface extending to the palatal pit; the caries did not affect the intact oblique ridge.

Radiographical Findings

Bite-wing radiograph shows moderate mesial and distal radiolucency.

Diagnosis: for tooth #26 is mesio-occlusodistal (MOD) caries lesion and intact oblique ridge.

Treatment: Two separate cavities; Class II MOD amalgam or composite restoration.

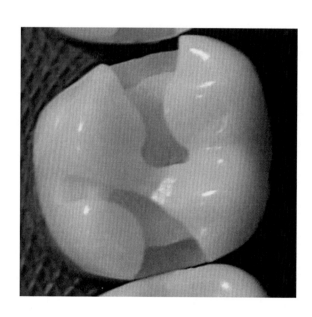

Ideal depth
1.5–2 mm

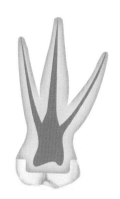

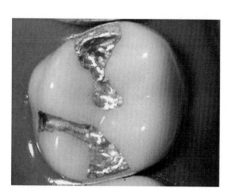

Ideal width
1-1.5mm or as
caries extends

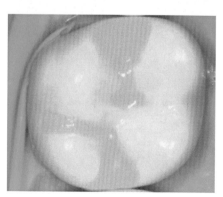

Task No. 11

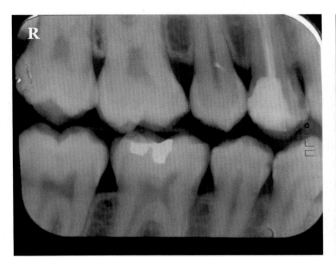 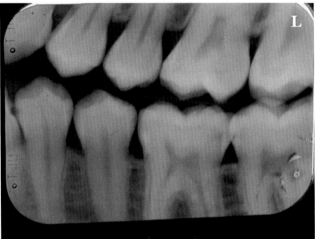

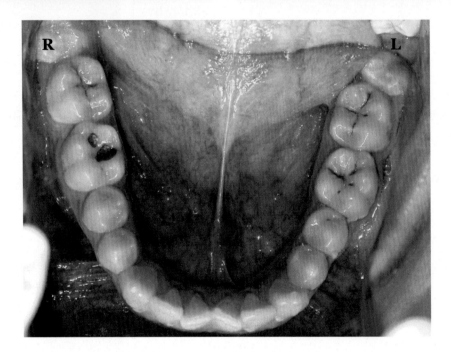

Patient Complaint
Periodic checkup for my teeth. No pain.

What is the clinical diagnosis for tooth #45?
What is the expected dental treatment for this case?

Clinical Findings
Solid and intact occlusal surface.

Radiographical Findings
Bite-wing radiograph shows small mesial radiolucency.

Diagnosis: for tooth #45 is mesial caries only.
Treatment: Mesial box only class II amalgam or composite restoration.

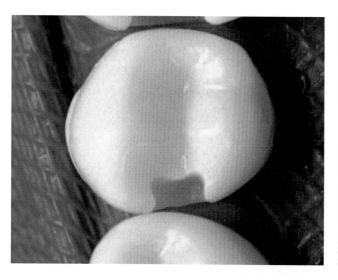
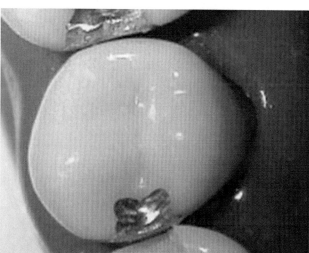
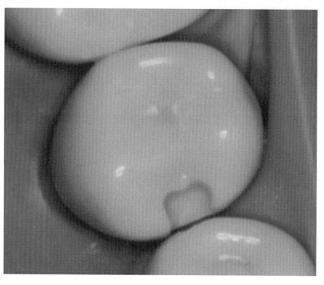
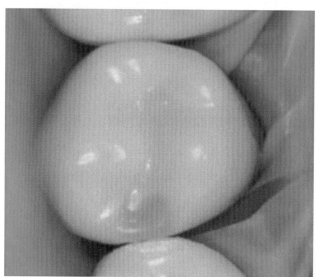

Task No. 12

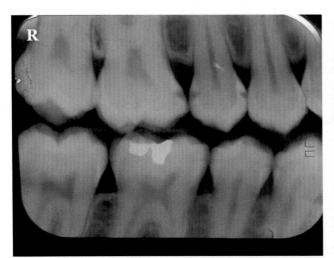
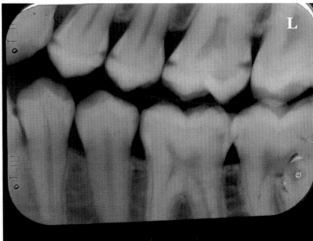
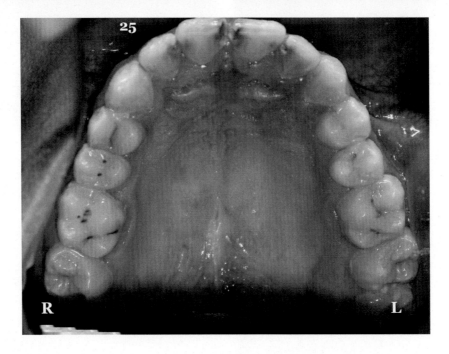

Patient Complaint
Periodic checkup for my teeth. No pain.

What is the clinical diagnosis for tooth #25?
What is the expected dental treatment for this case?

Clinical Findings
Slight black discolouration related to the mesial occlusal pit to tooth #25.

Radiographical Findings
Bite-wing radiograph shows small mesial radiolucency.

Diagnosis: **for tooth #25 is occlusomesial caries.**
Treatment: **occlusomesial class II amalgam or composite restoration.**

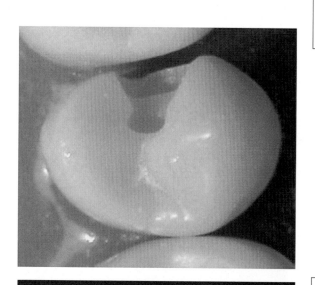

#25 OM intact transverse ridge

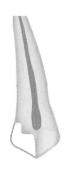

Ideal depth
1.5–2 mm

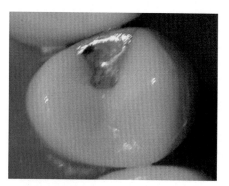

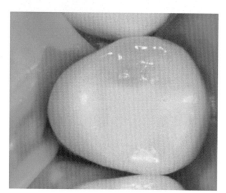

Ideal width
1-1.5mm or as
caries extends

Task No.13

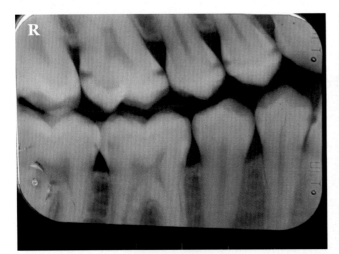 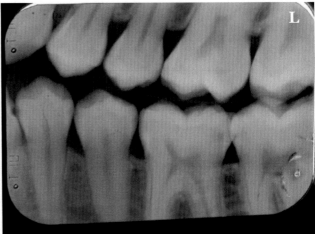

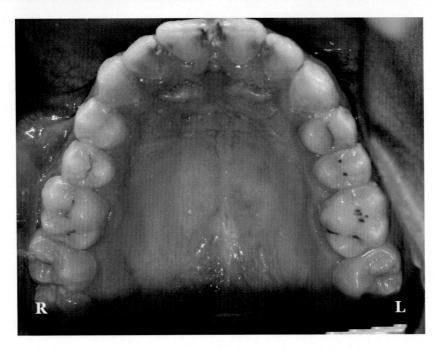

Patient Complaint
Slight pain with sweet food and cold drinks related to tooth # 15.

What is the clinical diagnosis for tooth #15?
What is the expected intervention to this case?

Clinical Findings

Small black discolouration in the occlusal surface bordered with White spot lesions more opaque when dried and disappear when wet with water.

Radiographical Findings

bite-wing radiograph shows small mesial radiolucency.

Diagnosis: for tooth #15 is occlusomesial caries.
Treatment: Occlusomesial class II amalgam or composite restoration

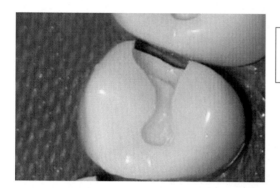

Ideal depth
1.5–2 mm

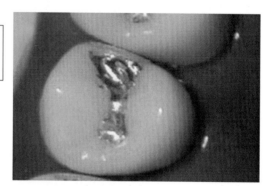

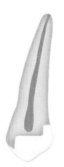

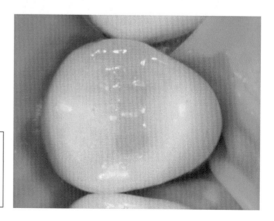

Ideal width
1-1.5mm or as
caries extends

Task No. 14

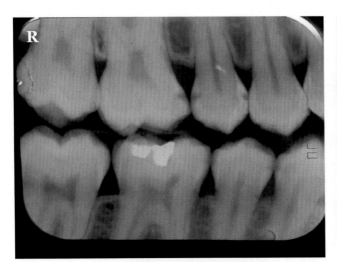
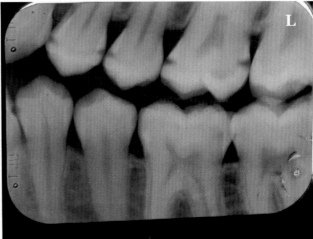
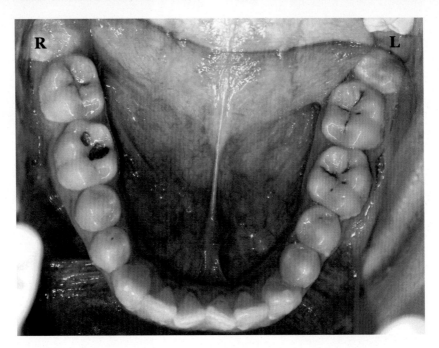

Patient Complaint
periodic checkup for my teeth. No pain.

What is the clinical diagnosis for tooth #44?
What is the expected dental treatment for this case?

Clinical Findings
slight black discolouration in distal occlusal
pit #44 not crossing the transverse ridge.

Radiographical Findings
bite-wing radiograph shows small distal radiolucency.

Diagnosis: for tooth #44 is occlusodistal caries and intact transverse ridge.
Treatment: occlusodistal class II amalgam or composite restoration.

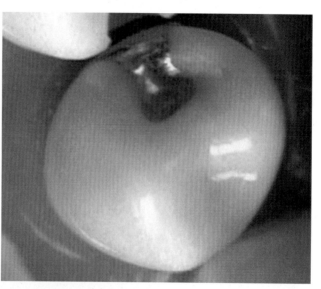

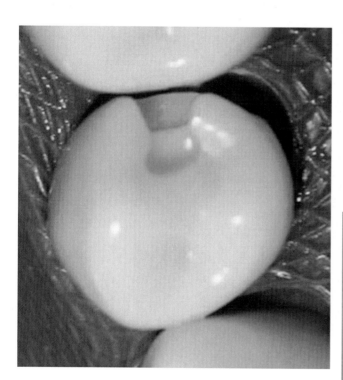

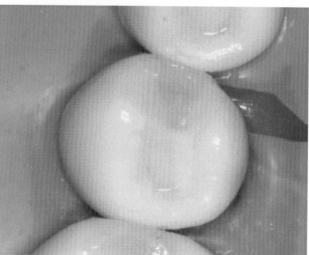

Task No. 15

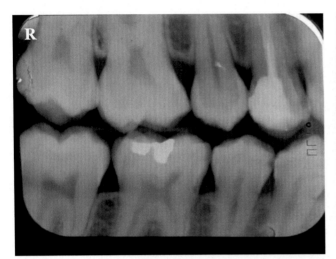
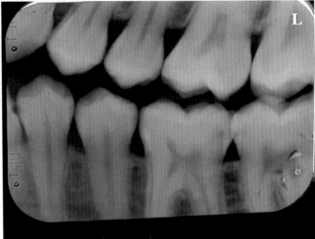

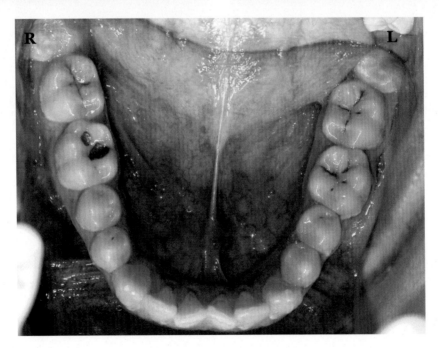

Patient Complaint
periodic checkup for my teeth. No pain.

What is the clinical diagnosis for tooth #45?
What is the expected dental treatment for this case?

Clinical Findings
slight black occlusal discolouration #45.

Radiographical Findings
bite-wing radiograph shows small mesial radiolucency.

Diagnosis: for tooth #45 is occlusomesial caries.
Treatment: occlusomesial class II amalgam or composite restoration.

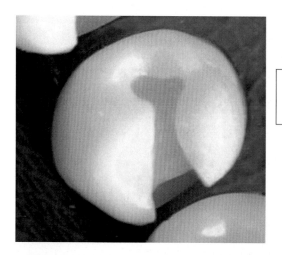

Ideal depth
1.5–2 mm

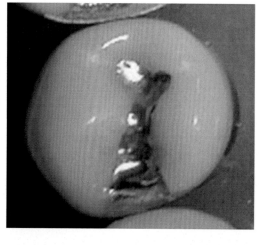

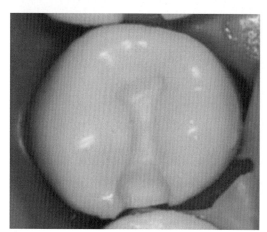

Ideal width
1-1.5mm or as
caries extends

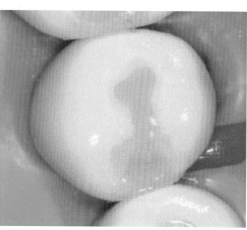

Task No. 16

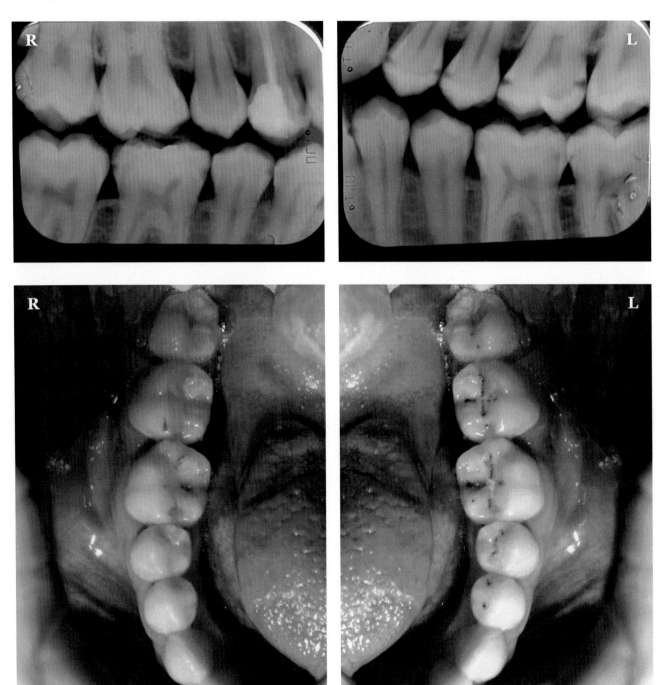

Patient Complaint
slight pain with sweet food and cold drinks related to tooth #46.

What is the clinical diagnosis for tooth #46? What is the expected dental treatment for this case?

Clinical Findings
cavitated black occlusal discolouration.

Radiographical Findings
bite-wing radiograph shows small mesial and distal radiolucency.

Diagnosis: for tooth #46 is Mesio-occlusodistal caries.
Treatment: Class II MOD amalgam or composite restoration.

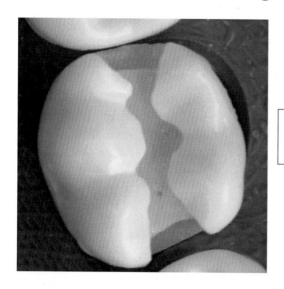

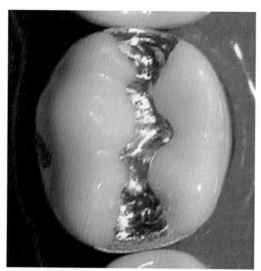

Ideal depth
1.5–2 mm

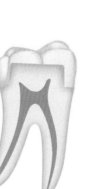

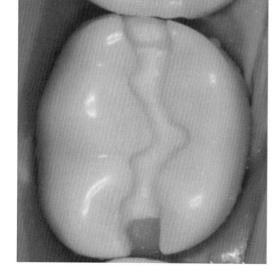

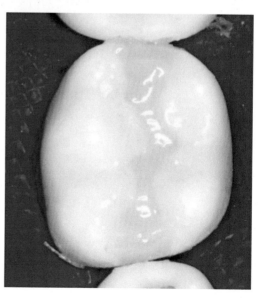

Ideal width
1-1.5mm or as
caries extends

Task No. 17

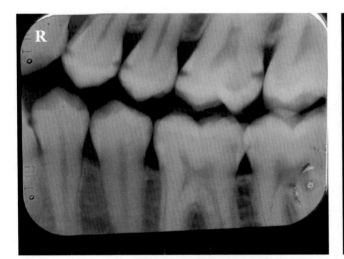
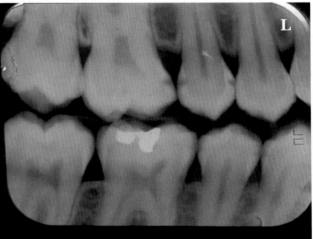

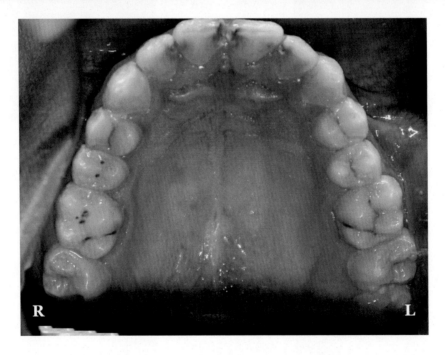

Patient Complaint
slight to moderate pain with sweet food
related to tooth #26.

What is the clinical diagnosis for tooth #26?
What is the expected dental treatment for this
case?

Clinical Findings

cavitated black occlusal discolouration crossing the oblique ridge.

Radiographical Findings

bite-wing radiograph shows small mesial and distal radiolucency.

Diagnosis: for tooth #26 is occlusomesial caries.
Treatment: occlusomesial (class II MO) amalgam or composite restoration.

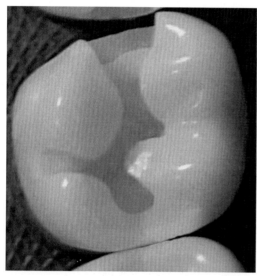

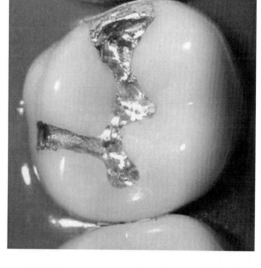

Ideal depth
1.5–2 mm

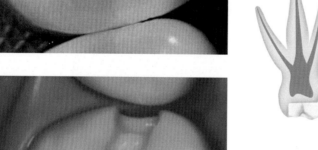

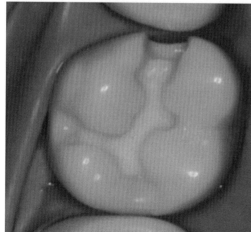

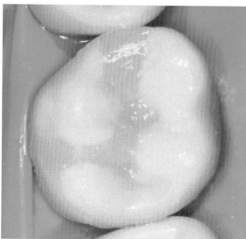

Ideal width
1-1.5mm or as
caries extends

Task No. 18

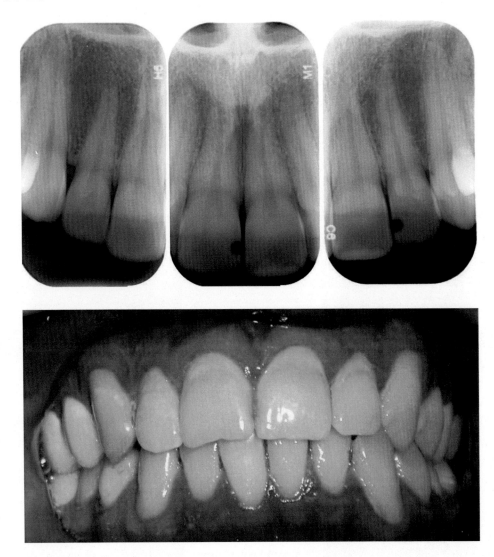

Patient Complaint
slight pain with cold drinks in the front teeth.

What is the clinical diagnosis for tooth #11?
What is the expected dental treatment for this case?

Clinical Findings

gray to black discolouration mesial of tooth #11 under transillumination with intact facial and lingual surface (with no cavitation).

Radiographical Findings

anterior periapical radiograph shows small to moderate mesial radiolucency of tooth #11.

Diagnosis: **for tooth #11 mesial caries.**
Treatment: **mesial (class III M) lingual approach composite restoration.**

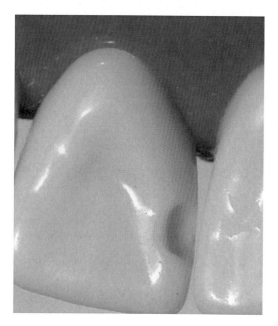 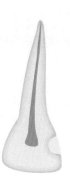 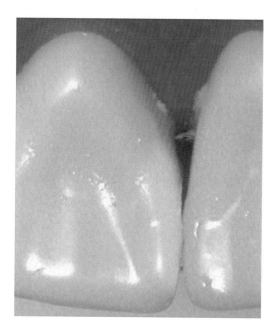

Task No. 19

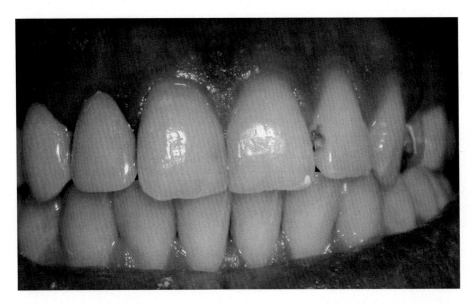 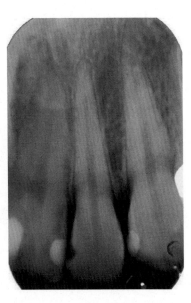

Patient Complaint
I want to restore my front tooth.

What is the clinical diagnosis for tooth #22?
What is the expected dental treatment for this case?

Clinical Findings
Cavitated facial gray to black discolouration mesial of tooth #22.

Radiographical Findings
anterior periapical radiograph shows moderate mesial radiolucency of tooth #22.

Diagnosis: for tooth #22 mesial caries.
Treatment: mesial (class III M) through-and-through approach composite restoration.

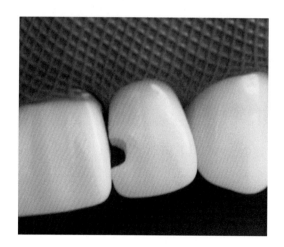
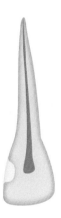
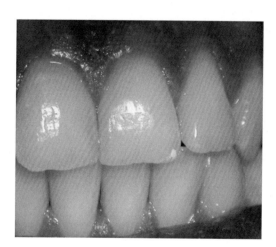

Task No. 20

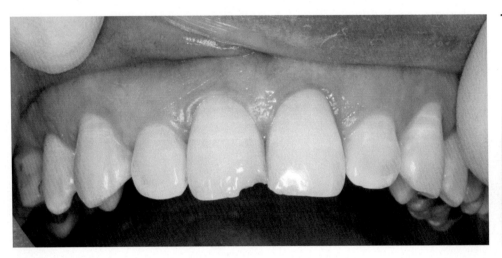 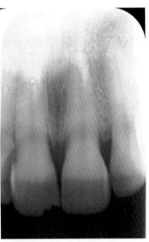

Complaint
part of my front tooth broke after eating hard nuts.

What is the clinical diagnosis for tooth #11?
What is the expected dental treatment for this case?

Clinical Findings

irregular fracture of the mesoincisal enamel corner of tooth #11

Radiographical Findings

no proximal caries only mesoincisal enamel fracture is clear in the periapical image.

Diagnosis: for tooth #11 mesoincisal enamel fracture class IV defect.
Treatment: class IV composite restoration.

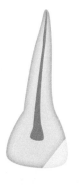

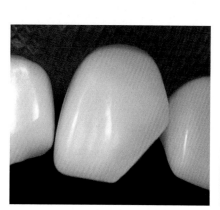
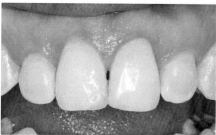
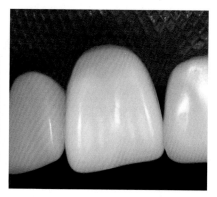

Task No. 21

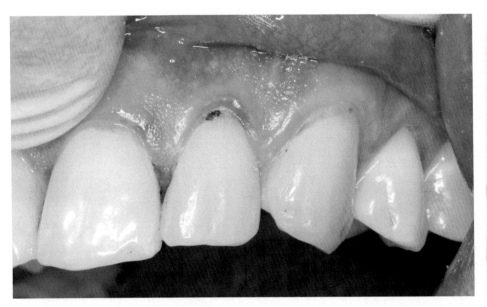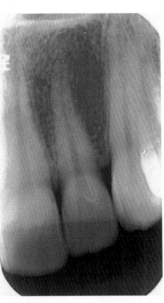

Patient Complaint
I want to restore my front tooth (points to tooth #22).

What is the clinical diagnosis for tooth #22?
What is the expected dental treatment for this case?

Clinical Findings
Black cavity cervical to tooth #22.

Radiographical Findings
no proximal caries.

Diagnosis: for tooth #22 facial cervical caries lesion.
Treatment: class V composite restoration.

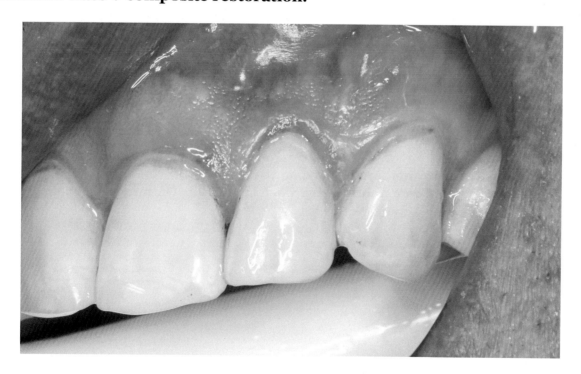

REFERENCES

1. Banerjee, Avijit, Watson, Timothy F. (2015), *Pickard's Guide to Minimally Invasive Operative Dentistry*, 10th edition, Oxford Medical Publication.
2. Heymann, Harald O., Swift, Edward J., and Ritter, Andre V. (2013), *Sturdevant's Art & Science of Operative Dentistry*, 6th edition, Elsevier.
3. Garg, Nisha, Garg, Amit (2013), *Textbook of Operative Dentistry*, 2nd edition, Jaypee Brothers Medical Publishers.
4. Hilton, Thomas J., Ferracane, Jack L., Broome, James C. (2013), *Summitt's Fundamentals of Operative Dentistry: A Contemporary Approach*, 4th edition, Quintessence Publishing Co.

ABOUT THE AUTHOR

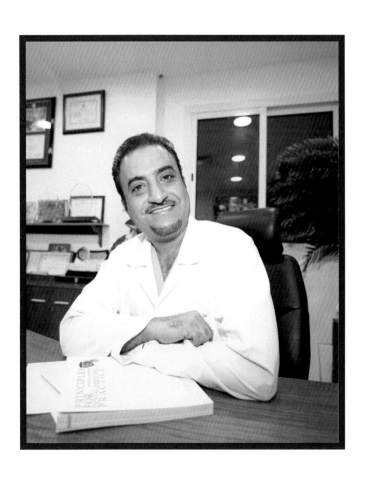

After graduating from King Saud University Dental College in 1996, Dr. Fahad Al-Qahtani (BDS, AEGD, ARD) has had a long career as a clinician and teacher.

Dr. Al-Qahtani taught undergraduate dental students in Riyadh Dental College from 2006 till 2014, using phantom lab courses, and participated in postgraduate programs for the Saudi Commission for Health Specialties and the Ministry of Health.

He always delivers his experience to his students in an easy, direct, and practical way.

Printed in the United States
By Bookmasters